Physiological Principles in Medicine:

a series of texts for medical students

General Editors

Dr R. N. Hardy
Physiological Laboratory, Cambridge

Professor M. Hobsley
Department of Surgical Studies, The Middlesex Hospital and the
Middlesex Hospital Medical School, London

Professor K. B. Saunders
Department of Medicine, St. George's Hospital and the St. George's
Hospital Medical School, London

Endocrine Physiology

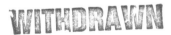

Physiological Principles in Medicine

Endocrine Physiology

Richard N. Hardy

Lecturer in Physiology, University of Cambridge;
Fellow and Tutor of Fitzwilliam College, Cambridge

Edward Arnold

A division of Hodder & Stoughton

LONDON   BALTIMORE   MELBOURNE   AUCKLAND

First published in Great Britain 1981
Fourth Impression 1988

British Library Cataloguing Publication Data

Hardy, Richard Neville
  Endocrine physiology. – (Physiological
  principles in medicine ISSN 0260-2946).
  1. Endocrine glands
  I. Title   II. Series
  616'.4   QP187
  ISBN 0 – 7131 – 4378 – 9
  ISSN 0260 – 2946

Whilst the advice and information in this book is believed to be true and
accurate at the date of going to press, neither the authors nor the
publisher can accept any legal responsibility or liability for any error or
omissions made.

Typeset in Compugraphic Baskerville by Reproduction Drawings Ltd
Printed and bound in Great Britain for Edward Arnold, the educational,
academic and medical publishing division of Hodder and Stoughton
Limited, 41 Bedford Square, London WC1B 3DQ
by J. W. Arrowsmith Ltd, Bristol

General preface to series

Student textbooks of medicine seek to present the subject of human diseases and their treatment in a manner that is not only informative, but interesting and readily assimilable. It is also important, in a field where knowledge advances rapidly, that the principles are emphasized rather than details, so that information remains valid for as long as possible.

These factors all favour an approach which concentrates on each disease as a disturbance of normal structure and function. Therapy, in principle, follows logically from a knowledge of the disturbance, though it is in this field that the most rapid changes in information occur.

A disturbance of normal structure without any disturbance of function is not important to the patient except for cosmetic or psychological considerations. Therefore, it is the disturbance in function which should be stressed. Preclinical students must get a firm grasp of physiology in a way that shows them how it is related to disease, while clinical students must be presented with descriptions of disease which stress the basic disturbance of function that is responsible for symptoms and signs. This approach should increase interest, reduce the burden on the student's memory and remain valid despite alterations in the details of treatment, so long as the fundamental physiological concepts remain unchallenged.

In the present Series, the major physiological systems are each covered by a pair of books, one preclinical and one clinical, in which the authors have attempted to meet the requirements discussed above. A particular feature is the provision of cross-references between the two members of a pair of books to facilitate the blending of basic science and clinical expertise that is the goal of this Series.

RNH
MH
KBS

Preface

This book is intended as an introduction to the study of endocrinology and has been written with the needs of preclinical medical students in mind. It therefore aims to provide a readable and up-to-date account of the endocrine system sufficient for candidates for the 2nd MB Examination or its equivalent. In addition, care has been taken to include (generally in smaller print) material beyond this level, notably in those parts of the subject which are advancing rapidly: for this reason it is hoped that the book will commend itself to honours students in physiology. The endocrinology of reproduction is not discussed in detail in this text but will be considered in the proposed two volumes on reproductive physiology in this Series.

Reference to endocrine disease has been restricted, since this topic forms the basis for the complementary book on clinical endocrinology in this Series and correspondingly, the clinical text will assume a basic knowledge of normal endocrine function.

I would like to express my thanks to Dr Peter Daggett, to my fellow General Editors and to my many colleagues in the Physiological Laboratory for their advice during the preparation of this text and in particular to Dr A. V. Edwards who was very largely responsible for writing Chapters 4 and 9. It would be invidious to single out any of the many secretaries in the Physiological Laboratory and Fitzwilliam College who have assisted with the typescript during the prolonged gestation of this book: I am extremely grateful to all of them for their patience and good humour. Finally, I am greatly indebted to Fiona Hake and Peter Starling for their skill in preparing the draft illustrations and to my publishers for their advice and encouragement.

Cambridge, 1981   RNH

Contents

Notes on the arrangement of this book

In a text of this length it is clearly impossible to describe the experimental basis of every assumption, but examples of evidence from a variety of experimental techniques have been included where appropriate. Liberal use has been made of figures and tables and, for ease of reference and, it is hoped, comprehension, each hormone/endocrine gland is discussed in the following standard sequence.

Anatomy and microstructure of the gland
Chemistry and metabolism of the hormone
Action of the hormone on the target cells
Effects of hormone deficiency
Effects of hormone excess
Control of hormone secretion.

The second section of the book contains a discussion of the coordinated behaviour of the components of the endocrine system in the control of energy metabolism and calcium homeostasis. Throughout the book it has been assumed that the reader has a working knowledge of basic biochemistry and, similarly, no attempt has been made to include detailed histological material.

Relation to Daggett: *Clinical Endocrinology*

This present book was written in conjunction with the corresponding clinical text, called *Clinical Endocrinology,* by Peter Daggett, and the two books have been planned to complement each other, as have other pairs of books in the *Physiological Principles in Medicine Series.* Thus, this book does not contain a detailed consideration of endocrine diseases and the clinical book assumes a knowledge of basic physiology.

Although each of the books will stand on its own, they are both designed to interdigitate with each other, and therefore each contains cross-referencing to the other. So, for example, if readers of this text wish to find out more about hyperparathyroidism (p.15), they will find a reference to the appropriate chapter in the clinical text, designated thus (Daggett: *Clinical Endocrinology,* Chapter 7). Similarly, references from the clinical book to this book will be designated (Hardy: *Endocrine Physiology,* Chapter 2).

References

Two types of references will be found in this book. First, at the end of this section, a list of General references, which are texts recommended for further general reading. Second, a list of Further reading as a general rule at the ends of the other chapters. Here reference will be made to recent reviews, monographs and occasionally original papers, to which the reader may refer in order to explore more deeply the material covered in that particular chapter.

General references

Bentley, P. J. (1976). *Comparative Vertebrate Endocrinology.* Cambridge University Press, London.

Bondy, P. K. and Rosenberg, L. E. (1980). *Metabolic Control and Disease.* W. B. Saunders, London.

Daggett, Peter (1981). *Clinical Endocrinology.* Edward Arnold, London.

Donovan, B. T. (1970). *Mammalian Endocrinology.* McGraw-Hill, London.

Ganong, W. F. (1979). *Review of Medical Physiology,* 9th edn. Lange, Los Altos.

Ganong, W. F. and Martini, L. (Eds.) (1973). *Frontiers in Neuroendocrinology.* Oxford University Press, New York.

Ganong, W. F. and Martini, L. (Eds.) (1978). *Frontiers in Neuroendocrinology,* Vol. V. Raven Press, New York.

Gray, C. H. and James, V. H. T. (1979). *Hormones in Blood,* Vol. III, 3rd edn. Academic Press, London.

Guyton, A. C. and McCann, S. M. (Eds.) (1974). *Endocrine Physiology.* MTP International Review of Science, Physiology, Series I, Vol. 5. Butterworths, London.

Guyton, A. C. and McCann, S. M. (Eds.) (1977). *Endocrine Physiology II.* International Review of Physiology Series, Vol. 16. University Park Press, Baltimore.

Martin, C. R. (1976). *Textbook of Endocrine Physiology.* Williams and Wilkins Co., Baltimore.

Martini, L. and Ganong, W. F. (Eds.) (1976). Frontiers in Neuro-endocrinology, Vol. IV. Raven Press, New York.

Parsons, J. A. (Ed.) (1976). *Peptide Hormones.* Macmillan Press, London.

Porter, R. and Fitzsimons, D. W. (Eds.) (1976). *Polypeptide Hormones: Molecular and Cellular Aspects.* Elsevier, Amsterdam.

Tepperman, J. (1973). *Metabolic and Endocrine Physiology,* 3rd edn. Year Book Medical Publishers, Chicago.

William, R. H. (Ed.) (1974). *Textbook of Endocrinology,* 5th edn. W. B. Saunders, Philadelphia.

Valuable review articles can also be found in:
Recent Progress in Hormone Research
Annual Review of Physiology
Physiological Reviews

1

Introduction

Communication between cells

One of the more obvious advantages possessed by multicellular organisms is the ability to differentiate cells which can perform particular and disparate functions and thereby increase the versatility of the organism as a whole. However, the presence of a variety of functionally adapted cell types necessitates the development of an efficient means of internal communication in order to coordinate and regulate their many activities.

There are basically only four ways in which one cell can influence the activity of another. Perhaps the most obvious method by which cells communicate with other cells in distant parts of the body is by means of cellular information channels called nerves, along which a frequency-modulated series of electrical changes, called nerve impulses, is directed between particular cells along precisely defined nerve fibres. In this communication system the specificity of the message is determined by the way in which the 'wiring diagram' is laid down, consequently it is sometimes called an 'anatomically addressed' system.

The three remaining types of communication involve the release of chemicals and may be considered to be 'chemically addressed' systems. The first, and simplest of these systems functions by virtue of close proximity: all cells affect their immediate neighbours non-specifically by consuming oxygen or metabolites from the interstitial fluid and releasing carbon dioxide or other products into it; such changes are incidental to general metabolism and probably serve no regulatory function. However, in the second case, certain cells influence their neighbours by the release of specific chemicals into the surrounding interstitial fluid which have *local* effects restricted to cells within a very small radius—such effects are called **paracrine** actions. Paracrine control is probably particularly important in the alimentary tract but, because technical difficulties make it a difficult field to study, paracrine physiology is still in its infancy.

This book is concerned with the final type of intercellular communication, termed **endocrine**, in which cells influence other cells by releasing into the circulating body fluid particular chemicals called hormones, which, although carried into contact with every cell in the body, only affect those **target cells** which possess particular recognition features (hormone receptors).

Ignoring paracrine control, the two main executive control systems, nerves

1

and hormones, both appeared early in evolutionary development. To an extent this is not altogether surprising since, in general terms, each system subserves a different mode of control. Thus, nerves assume importance where a fast, rapidly modulated control channel is required, such as for example that which initiates and coordinates voluntary movement. Hormones, conversely, would seem best adapted for longer-term regulation, where speed of response and continuous rapid variation are of secondary importance to a stable, prolonged regulatory action. However, such a rigid segregation of nervous and endocrine control pathways as that above would now be considered naive, in view of the mass of evidence available to indicate the many ways in which the two systems can be seen to act *in concert;* research into aspects of **neuroendocrinology** accounts for the vast majority of current work on the endocrine system.

The concept of a hormone

What is a hormone? A simple question to which there is no simple, 'watertight' answer, for it is extremely difficult to devise a precise, succinct definition of a hormone which includes all those compounds generally held to be hormones while excluding all those which are not. Most working definitions are variations on the following general theme. 'A hormone is a substance secreted *directly into the blood* by discrete *specialized cells* (which may be grouped into an endocrine gland) in *response to a specific stimulus* (neural or bloodborne) and in amounts which *vary with the strength of the stimulus.* Hormones are present in only *minute concentrations* in blood and when carried to their *target cells* exert specific effects which always involve the *regulation of pre-existing cellular reactions* other than by the provision of metabolic energy.' This definition may seem unnecessarily cumbersome, but when you have read this book, try to do two things:

1. See if the definition fits all compounds assumed to be hormones;
2. See if it excludes all other possibilities, such as that CO_2 is a hormone produced by exercising muscle to stimulate respiration, or glucose is a hormone produced by the liver for the benefit of exercising muscle.

The history of endocrinology

The birth of endocrinology is generally accepted to be the classic paper by Bayliss and Starling (1902) in which they described secretin and analysed its actions on secretion from the denervated pancreas. They called secretin a 'chemical messenger' and it was left to a colleague, W. B. Hardy, to coin the word **hormone** from a greek verb meaning 'I excite to activity'. With the wisdom of hindsight, however, it is clear that many observations prior to 1902 can now be explained in endocrinological terms (Table 1.1).

As is almost always the case in science, advances in our understanding of the endocrine system have been largely secondary to improvements in experimental methodology. This is reflected in Table 1.1, which illustrates in chronological order some of the major landmarks in the development of the subject and should be studied with the content of Table 1.2 also in mind.

Table 1.1 The history of endocrinology

Early observations

From antiquity	Effects of castration on man and animals
1849	Testis transplant prevents atrophy of cock's comb after castration
1850	Cretinism associated with congenital absence of thyroid
1855	Adrenal malfunction in man (Addison's disease)
1869	Discovery of pancreatic islets
1886	Acromegaly in man (overproduction of growth hormone)

Major landmarks by decades

1890	Sheep thyroid grafts relieve myoedema in man
	Pressor agents extracted from posterior pituitary and adrenal
	Pancreatectomy produces diabetes in dog
	Parathyroidectomy produces tetany
1900	Isolation, purification and synthesis of adrenaline
	Action of secretin described
	First use of term 'hormone'
	Action of posterior pituitary extracts on kidney and uterus
1910	Effects of hypophysectomy described
	Diabetes insipidus controlled by posterior pituitary extracts
1920	Insulin prepared from pancreatic extracts
	Anterior pituitary hormones discovered
	Structure of thyroxine established; thyroxine synthesized
1930	Hypothalamo-pituitary portal system described
	Structure and synthesis of gonadal steroids and adrenal glucocorticoids
1940	Parathyroid secretion shown to be influenced by blood Ca^{2+}
	Mode of neural control of anterior pituitary analysed
1950	Amino acid sequence of insulin described
	Discovery of aldosterone
	Synthesis of oxytocin and vasopressin
1960	Competitive radio-immunoassays developed
	Calcitonin discovered
	Potency of vitamin D metabolites discovered
	Hypothalamic-releasing and -inhibiting hormones isolated
	TRH structure established and synthesis achieved
	Prostaglandin actions
	Role of cAMP in hormone action demonstrated
	Action of other hormones on genome defined
	Three-dimensional structure of insulin described
1970	Inter-relations of brain/gut peptides explored
	Endorphins and enkephalins discovered
	Endocrinology of fetus investigated
	Immunocytochemical localization of endocrine cells
	Role of calmodulin in intracellular regulation

The analysis of endocrine activity

In the case of most of the major endocrine glands, their identity has been uncovered by the appearance of a 'deficiency syndrome' as a result of decrease or failure in secretion of a particular hormone, brought about by disease or damage to the gland. Further analysis of the function of a newly discovered endocrine system usually follows the lines illustrated in Table 1.2. Needless to say, the complete 'dossier' envisaged in Table 1.2 is not yet available for every hormone and endocrine gland, but such comprehensive documentation is obviously the goal of endocrinological research.

Table 1.2   The experimental analysis of endocrine function

Basic evidence

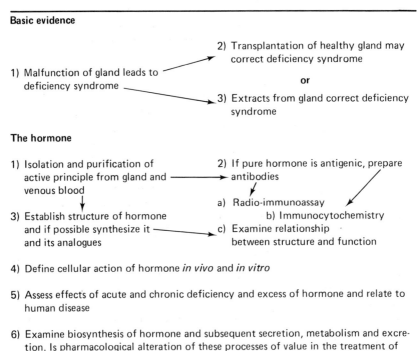

1) Malfunction of gland leads to deficiency syndrome

2) Transplantation of healthy gland may correct deficiency syndrome

or

3) Extracts from gland correct deficiency syndrome

The hormone

1) Isolation and purification of active principle from gland and venous blood

2) If pure hormone is antigenic, prepare antibodies

3) Establish structure of hormone and if possible synthesize it and its analogues

a) Radio-immunoassay
b) Immunocytochemistry
c) Examine relationship between structure and function

4) Define cellular action of hormone *in vivo* and *in vitro*

5) Assess effects of acute and chronic deficiency and excess of hormone and relate to human disease

6) Examine biosynthesis of hormone and subsequent secretion, metabolism and excretion. Is pharmacological alteration of these processes of value in the treatment of disease?

The endocrine gland

1) Macroscopic, microscopic and ultrastructural examination

2) Embryological origin and development of gland

3) Immunocytochemical localization of hormone and metabolites

4) Comparative study of gland in other mammalian species and phylogenetic analysis of structure and function if present in submammalian groups.

Table 1.2 continued

Analysis of possible control mechanisms

1) Control by nerves?
   a)   Examine effect of denervation or transplantation to a remote site
   b)   Look for nerves associated with secretory cells
   c)   Assess effect of electrical stimulation of nerves
   d)   Try pharmacological blockade

2) Control by bloodborne factors?
   a)   Look for direct effects on the gland of blood parameters influenced by the hormone (e.g. glucose, Ca^{2+}, volume)
   b)   Examine possible role of anterior pituitary by noting effects of hypophysectomy and pituitary extracts
   c)   Look for feedback effects of the hormone or its metabolites

3) The central nervous system (CNS)

If 1) or 2b) above yield positive results it is likely the CNS is implicated in control of the gland

   a)   Look for evidence for CNS involvement e.g. circadian pattern of secretion or relation to environmental factors such as stress, temperature or day length
   b)   Attempt detailed localization of the neural areas involved (usually in the hypothalamus) using stereotactic methods to destroy, stimulate or record from precisely defined areas

The cellular basis of hormone action

The problem of the mode of action of hormones on cells is still largely unresolved; moreover, any comprehensive discussion must assume a knowledge of biochemistry and familiarity with those endocrine systems from which convenient examples can be cited. For these reasons the following account makes no claim to be comprehensive: it will not assume other than a superficial knowledge of biochemistry and will leave the reader to consult other texts to pursue this aspect. We will, however, draw upon examples of hormone action discussed later in *this* text: reference will be made to the appropriate page, but the reader may wish to defer reading this section until *after* having studied later chapters.

Before examining how hormones can influence *individual cells,* it is worth noting that hormones can affect the functioning of specific *groups* of cells (tissues) in more general ways. These include stimulation of growth of the tissues by promoting an increase in the number of cells (this is often called a **trophic** effect) and increase in blood flow through the tissue due to a vasodilator effect on local blood vessels (e.g. ACTH promotes adrenal blood flow, p.118).

At the level of individual cells, hormones influence activity basically by controlling one or more rate-limiting steps in the metabolism of the cell. Almost without exception, such control devolves ultimately upon the production or activation of specific proteins, usually with enzyme activity. How this is achieved depends upon the chemical nature of the hormone involved, as illustrated in Fig. 1.1. The following account should be read in conjunction with Fig. 1.1 by reference to the numerical sequence.

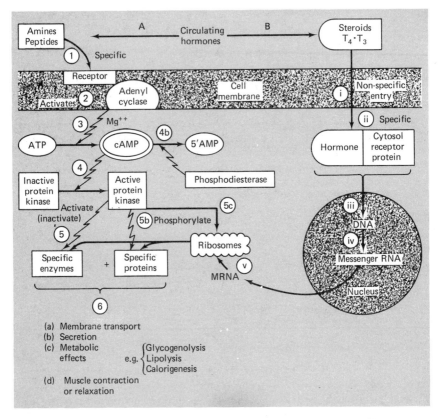

Fig. 1.1 Diagram to illustrate the basic pathways by which; A, amine and peptide hormones and B, steroid and thyroid hormones regulate the synthesis of specific proteins and thereby modulate cell function. For detailed explanation see text. ATP = adenosine triphosphate; AMP = adenosine monophosphate; cAMP = cyclic adenosine—$3'$, $5'$—monophosphate ('cyclic AMP'); T_4 = thyroxine, T_3 = triiodothyronine.

A. Amine and peptide hormones

1. These hormones do not enter the cells, but each reacts with a specific receptor in the cell membrane.

2. Combination with the receptor activates membrane-bound adenyl (adenylate) cyclase.

3. This enzyme, in the presence of Mg^{2+}, induces the formation, from ATP, of cyclic AMP (cAMP).

4. This nucleotide activates one or more of the cAMP-dependent protein kinases with the cell.

4b. The cAMP is degraded by phosphodiesterase producing $5'$AMP.

5. The active protein kinase promotes the phosphorylation of specific enzymes which may serve to activate, or sometimes deactivate, the enzyme.

5b. Phosphorylation may also alter the configuration and properties of other specific proteins (e.g. structural or membrane proteins).

5c. Active protein kinases may themselves activate protein synthesis at the ribosomal level.

6. The enzymes and other proteins influenced by the preceding events implement the final action on cell function (a–d in Fig. 1.1).

The above is a brief and general account of the '2nd messenger' concept originally formulated by Sutherland and co-workers in 1961, as a result of their analysis of the action of hormones on glycogen breakdown in liver cells, (the hormone outside the cell is the '1st messenger', cAMP within the cell is the '2nd messenger'). A more detailed discussion of the role of cAMP will be found in the sections on glucagon, p.39; catecholamines p.21; and ACTH p.117; Table 1.3 summarizes some of the more important hormone actions known to be mediated via cAMP.

It should be noted that some hormonal affects may be the result of a *decrease* in cAMP activity: these include some of the α effects of catecholamines (see Table 3.1) and the decrease in glycogenolysis and lipolysis brought about by insulin (see Fig. 4.7, and p.32).

Recent evidence suggests that cAMP may not be the only '2nd messenger' and attention is being focussed on the role of other nucleotides, particularly cyclic $3'-5'$ guanosine monophosphate (cyclic GMP). Evidence is also accumulating to implicate prostaglandins (p.144) in the intracellular mechanism of action of certain hormones.

Table 1.3 Some of the hormone actions mediated by cAMP mentioned later in this book.

Hormone	Tissue	Action	Ref. page
Adrenaline/noradrenaline	Liver Muscle Adipose tissue Heart	Glycogenolysis Glycogenolysis Lipolysis Positive inotropic action	22
Glucagon	Liver Adipose tissue Pancreas	Glycogenolysis Lipolysis Insulin secretion	40
ACTH	Adrenal cortex	Steroidogenesis	117
TSH	Thyroid	Increased secretion of T_4, T_3	105
Parathyroid hormone	Bone Kidney Intestine	Alters membrane permeability to Ca^{2+}	13
Arginine vasopressin (ADH)	Kidney	Increases water permeability	57
Hypothalamic-releasing hormones	Anterior pituitary	Increases secretion of hormones	71

B. Steroid hormones, thyroxine (T_4) and tri-iodothyronine (T_3) (see Fig. 1.1)

i. These hormones enter cells freely.

ii. They bind to specific receptor proteins within the cytosol.

iii. The hormone – receptor complex then passes into the nucleus, binds reversably with DNA and functions as a 'gene-activator' (transcription process).

iv. The appropriate messenger RNA (mRNA) is produced and leaves the nucleus.

v. The mRNA promotes the synthesis of specific proteins and enzymes within the ribosomes (translation process).

Understanding of the details of the cellular action of hormones has been aided by the existence of drugs which will enhance or inhibit various stages of the process. For example, cAMP-mediated actions are usually enhanced by methyl xanthines (e.g. theophylline, caffeine), which inhibit phospho-diesterase (Fig. 1.1, 4b). Similarly, the actions of steroid hormones may be investigated by blocking transcription (Fig. 1.1, iv), by actinomycin D, or translation (Fig. 1.1, v), by puromycin.

One very new and exciting field of research concerns the possible role of Ca^{2+}-binding proteins in the modulation of cellular metabolism *after* the actions of the 1st messenger (hormones) and 2nd messenger (cyclic nucleotides). A great many cell functions are regulated to a greater or lesser extent by Ca^{2+}, including cyclic nucleotide metabolism itself, cell motility, muscle contraction, chromosome movement, endocytosis, exocytosis, axonal flow and neuro-transmitter release. Recent work has revealed the existence of a specific Ca^{2+}-binding protein called **calmodulin,** which has been found in the cells of a wide variety of plant and animal tissues, from cotton-seed to bovine brain, to rat testis, to coelenterates! Calmodulin has been characterized and has 148 amino acids and a mol. wt. of 17 000. Its seemingly ubiquitous distribution in living cells (in the cytoplasm, but *not* the nucleus) argues in favour of it playing a pivotal role in the intracellular regulation of activity. Evidence is accumulating to indicate that calmodulin acts as a 'receptor' for Ca^{2+} such that, in order to become physiologically active, Ca^{2+} must first bind to calmodulin, or, in the case of muscle cells, to analagous proteins such as the troponins, which are in fact very similar in structure.

Measurement of hormones

Accurate estimation of the concentrations of particular hormones in blood or urine is a vital tool both to basic research and to the evaluation of endocrine disease. Ideally, an assay should combine the virtues of accuracy, specificity, sensitivity, simplicity and low cost, but it is only within the last decade that these objectives have been approached. Basically, assays can be divided into biological and chemical methods.

Biological assays (bioassays)

These rely upon the measurement of some index of the biological action of the hormone and can either involve a whole animal *(in vivo)* or an isolated organ, tissue or cell *(in vitro)*. A good example of an *in vivo* assay is the thyroid neck-counting method (see Fig. 8.5), an example of an *in vitro* method would be the measurement of TSH from its promotion of the uptake of iodide by thyroid slices. While perhaps more 'physiological', in the sense that the measurement is of biological activity rather than a chemical property, biological assays are generally cumbersome, expensive and time consuming.

Chemical methods

General chemical methods
Since hormones have a specific molecular structure, they can be detected and measured by several techniques which depend on their molecular configuration. The most specific is gas-liquid chromatography combined with mass-spectography.

Less specific methods depend upon the ability of the molecule to produce fluorescence under particular conditions, or to be converted to a coloured compound by a chemical reaction. The catecholamines (adrenaline and noradrenaline) can be converted into fluorescent compounds, for instance. If these techniques are combined with separative measures, such as thin-layer or column chromatography, a high degree of specificity can be achieved. Thus, although most steroids fluoresce, progesterone can be assayed quite effectively by extraction into ether, which leaves many other steroids in the aqueous phase, and then column chromatography on a gel (Sephadex LH 20), which separates progesterone from other interfering steroids which would also fluoresce.

Saturation analysis
In recent years, systems which depend upon the ability of certain molecules to bind hormones in a reversible fashion have been adapted for measuring hormones. If a compound X will bind a hormone H, in the presence of a fixed amount of X an equilibrium will exist, in which some H is bound to X and some H is free; the exact proportions depending on the amount of H.

Principle

$$X \quad + \quad H \quad \rightleftharpoons \quad X \sim H$$

Binding agent   Hormone   Bound complex

Method If a very small amount of radioactively labelled hormone (H^*) is first added to the binding agent, so that nearly all the hormone is bound, the equilibrium will be well across to the right. The labelled hormone is usually referred to as 'hot' hormone.

$$\text{X} \quad + \quad \text{H}^* \quad \underset{\longleftarrow}{\overset{\longrightarrow}{\rule{2cm}{0pt}}} \quad \text{X} \sim \text{H}^*$$

Fixed quantity of binding agent	Trace amount of 'hot' hormone	Bound, 'hot' hormone — effectively 100 per cent of the added 'hot' hormone

If now 'cold' hormone (H), either a standard or sample, is added, it will compete with the 'hot' hormone for the limited number of binding sites.

$$\text{X} \quad + \quad \underbrace{\text{H} \quad + \quad \text{H}^*}_{\text{Total free hormone}} \quad \rightleftharpoons \quad \underbrace{\text{X} \sim \text{H}^* \quad + \quad \text{X} \sim \text{H}}_{\text{Total bound hormone}}$$

Obviously, as more H is added, since the amount of X, the binding agent, is fixed, the proportion of H^* which will be bound will decrease. Thus a standard curve can be obtained which shows the amount of 'cold' hormone in the sample from the progressive decrease in the amount of 'hot' hormone bound.

Three major types of binding agent are used.

1. Antibodies—these have to be produced for each hormone as required. These are referred to as radio-immunoassays (RIA) and can be used for any hormone to which an antibody can be prepared. Radio-immunoassays can now be used even for hormones such as steroids, which are not usually themselves antigenic, by binding the hormone to an antigenic molecule such as serum albumen: specific antibody is then produced against the complex.

2. Plasma proteins which normally bind the hormone as it circulates. These are readily available by taking blood from an animal. These are referred to as protein-binding assays.

3. Tissue receptors—these can be extracted and concentrated from the tissue which normally responds to the hormone, since the first step in hormone action appears to be the binding of the hormone to the cell membrane. This type of assay is referred to as a receptor assay.

The importance of the development of saturation analysis methods since the pioneer work of Ekins, and also that of Berson and Yalow, cannot be overstated: without such assays, progress in endocrine research in the past fifteen years would have been very substantially reduced.

Further reading

Daggett, Peter (1981). *Clinical Endocrinology.* Edward Arnold, London.

Sönksen, P. H. (Ed.) (1974). Radioimmunoassay and saturation analysis. *British Medical Bulletin* **30**, 1.

Sutherland, E. W. (1972). Studies on the mechanism of hormone action. *Science* **177**, 401.

Unit 12. Hormones and Receptors. (1977). Open University Press, Milton Keynes.

2

The parathyroid gland

The parathyroid glands are found in the neck and secrete the polypeptide hormone parathormone (PTH) which is involved in calcium homeostasis.

Anatomy and microstructure

In man there are usually four parathyroid glands. They are small structures, oval in shape, weighing some 30 to 40 mg each and are found close to the dorsal surface of the thyroid gland (Fig. 2.1). Both the superior and inferior pairs of parathyroids are supplied by the inferior thyroid artery. Rarely, five or even six glands are found and some may be found within the mediastinum as far down as aortic arch.

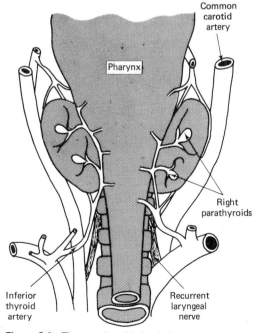

Figure 2.1 The parathyroid glands in man, seen from behind.

Histologically, the glands are seen to have a rich blood supply and to comprise two types of secretory cell: the 'chief' cells are relatively small with cytoplasmic vacuoles, the 'oxyphil' cells are less common, larger, and have granules within the cytoplasm which stain with eosin. Parathormone (PTH) is secreted by the 'chief' cells: the function of the 'oxyphil' cells remains uncertain, but they are not present before puberty.

Chemistry and metabolism of parathormone

Parathormone is an acid polypeptide containing 84 amino acids (Fig. 2.2). The biological activity appears to reside within the first 20 to 29 amino acids of the chain.

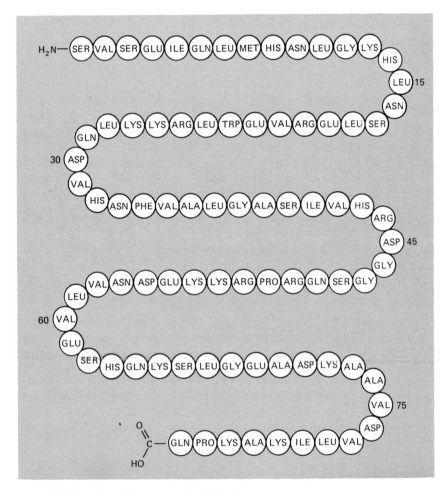

Figure 2.2 Structure of human parathyroid hormone.

It is now known that at least three molecular cleavages occur between the initial synthesis and the disappearance from the circulation. The gland first synthesizes pre-pro-PTH, containing at least 115 amino acids. This is cleaved to produce pro-PTH, with 90 amino acids (approximate mol. wt. 12 000), which enters the storage granules and is then converted to PTH (mol. wt. 9500) before release into the circulation. Subsequently, a second cleavage results in a large inactive fragment (mol. wt. 7000) and a smaller fragment (mol. wt. 2500) of uncertain biological effects. Much current research is directed toward an evaluation of the significance of these molecular cleavages, since the diverse actions of PTH on bone, kidney and gut described below may be explicable in terms of molecular fragmentation. Such studies are hampered by technical problems inherent in the detection and accurate measurement of the concentration of the various PTH fragments within the blood.

Actions of parathormone on target tissues

Parathormone has three principal actions, each of which helps to increase the blood calcium concentration (hypercalcaemic effects).

Effect on bone

Parathormone promotes the resorption of bone, thereby mobilizing calcium and phosphate. Details of this action remain unclear, although it appears to involve increased formation of cAMP. The dissolution of bone depends in part on the stimulation of lysosymal enzymes within osteocytes (osteolysis) and osteoclasts (osteoclasis), thereby breaking down the organic matrix of the bone, as evidenced by the increased excretion of hydroxyproline—an amino acid present in high concentration in the collagen. This action of PTH on bone is extremely rapid and concurrent with a local decrease in pH resulting from increased citrate and lactate production from the tissue. Associated with the physical degradation of the bone, there is an increase in the phagocytic action of osteoclasts, while osteoblast activity is depressed. In the longer term more osteoclasts are formed.

Effect on the kidney

Parathormone facilitates the reabsorption of the calcium and depresses the reabsorption of phosphate by kidney tubules. The first of these actions is less important, and indeed a reduction of calcium clearance has not been demonstrated in all species studied. However, the decrease in phosphate reabsorption (phosphaturic effect) is well established and extremely important. Micropuncture studies have shown that PTH depresses the reabsorption of both phosphate and sodium by the proximal tubule. It has been suggested that the hormone acts via cAMP to inhibit sodium reabsorption, and that the depression of phosphate reabsorption is secondary to this. In practice, the extra sodium remaining in the tubule is reabsorbed distally so the PTH does not cause natiuresis, whereas little, if any, phosphate is absorbed beyond the proximal tubule so that a pronounced phosphaturia results. This increased renal excretion of phosphate serves to reduce plasma phosphate concentration. Since calcium and phosphate have a solubility product relationship, such that the product of the concentration of the free ions remains constant, the fall in blood phosphate which results from the increased renal excretion necessitates increased entry of calcium from bone into the blood to maintain the solubility product.

There is no doubt that the actions of PTH on bone and the kidney both contribute to the overall hypercalcaemic action of this hormone, but it is difficult to assess which is more important in quantitative terms.

Effect on the intestine

Parathormone is said to enhance the absorption of calcium from the intestine. However, vitamin D and certain of its metabolites facilitate calcium absorption to a much greater extent: this led to the idea that the contribution of PTH was of relatively little significance. Recently, however, work has shown that PTH probably influences the conversion within the kidney of hydroxylated vitamin D (25-hydroxycholecalciferol, p.157) to the dihydroxylated metabolite (1,25-dihydroxycholecalciferol) which is much more effective in promoting intestinal calcium absorption. If this is indeed the case, the PTH assumes considerably more importance in the control of calcium absorption, albeit in an indirect way.

Effects of parathormone deficiency (hypoparathyroidism)

Parathormone is essential for life; if the parathyroid glands are removed, there is a gradual decrease in plasma calcium which, if uncorrected, results in a progressive increase in neuromuscular excitability leading to tetany and death.

> At first sight it may seem paradoxical that a *decrease* in blood calcium leads to muscular spasm, particularly when it is remembered that calcium ions are essential for the release of acetyl choline from motor end–plates and also play a vital role in excitation–contraction coupling within the muscles: for these reasons a decrease in blood calcium might be expected to result in impairment of muscular contraction. The explanation is that during a gradual *decline* in blood calcium concentration (progressive hypocalcaemia) the first effect is on motor pathways within the CNS such as to cause a spontaneous and repetitive discharge of impulses. These impulses promote the tetanic contractions: blood calcium concentration must fall much further before neuromuscular block ensues or excitation–contraction coupling is impaired. In practice, if no treatment is given, the tetanic contractions, which initially involve only the hands, feet and face, become more generalized and the patient eventually succumbs to laryngeal spasm leading to asphyxiation. Thus, in life, the blood calcium never falls to levels low enough to cause neuromuscular block or failure of excitation–contraction coupling.

The acute consequences of total removal of PTH are most commonly encountered in patients following either accidental removal of the parathyroids or damage to their blood supply during operations on the neck, notably thyroidectomy or radical dissection to remove malignant tissue (Daggett: *Clinical Endocrinology*, Chapter 7). Under these circumstances, tetany usually occurs within a few days postoperatively and is sometimes associated with mental symptoms such as psychosis. Such patients are treated in the first instance by measures directed toward restoring normal blood calcium concentrations, such as a slow intravenous infusion of calcium gluconate. Thereafter, treatment involves the facilitation of intestinal calcium absorption by the administration of vitamin D_3 or a derivative and by oral calcium supplementation. Parathormone therapy cannot be used as a long-term measure as, for some reason, it loses its effect after a few weeks.

Hypoparathyroidism is also found rarely in cases of congenital absence or underdevelopment (hypoplasia) of the glands: this may also be associated with agenesis of the thymus gland (Di George syndrome). In the former case, serious symptoms of parathyroid deficiency may not manifest themselves until relatively late in life. In the Di George syndrome, however, the patients usually die in infancy of infection secondary to immunodeficiency.

Tetany is occasionally encountered in newborn infants, usually within the first week of life. It is most common in premature infants which are fed on cows' milk and is probably the result of immaturity of the parathyroid glands exacerbated by the high ratio of phosphate to calcium in bovine milk. Maternal hyperparathyroidism also predisposes the newborn to tetany as a consequence of the suppression of the infant's own parathyroids, although in such cases the hypoparathyroidism is usually of short duration.

Pseudohypoparathyroidism is a rare hereditary disorder in which the symptoms of hypoparathyroidism are present despite the fact that parathyroid secretion is excessive and the parathyroid glands show signs of hyperplasia. In this disease, the target tissues—bone and kidney—appear to be extremely resistant to the actions of PTH, possibly due to a failure in stimulation of membrane-bound adenyl cyclase. Needless to say, this condition cannot be treated by PTH administration.

Effects of parathormone excess (primary hyperparathyroidism)

Oversecretion of PTH results in abnormally high blood calcium levels associated with lowered blood phosphate levels (hypophosphataemia). Renal calcium excretion is elevated due to increased glomerular filtration of calcium and often results in the formation of kidney stones. Demineralization of bones of varying degrees of severity is often found. In man, hyperparathyroidism is usually the result of the presence of a benign tumour (adenoma) of one, or rarely several, of the parathyroid glands: carcinoma of the parathyroid gland is rare (Daggett: *Clinical Endocrinology,* Chapter 7).

The skeletal changes in hyperparathyroidism show wide variations between subjects. Many patients have no obvious bone disease, while others may show signs of generalized decalcification and sometimes the formation of bone cysts (osteitis fibrosa cystica) or giant cell pseudotumours consisting mainly of osteoclasts (osteoclastomas). Renal changes are the consequence of the excessive filtration of calcium and involve both the formation of calcium-rich calculi and also general calcification of the tubular cells. Severely impaired renal function may result from these changes and is the most usual cause of death in this condition.

Surgical removal of the affected gland usually results in a dramatic reversal of the symptoms.

Control of parathormone secretion

Parathormone secretion is controlled by a direct feedback effect of ionized calcium on the parathyroid; increase in ionized calcium depresses PTH secretion; conversely, secretion is stimulated by a fall in ionized calcium (Fig. 2.3). Calcium ions may decrease PTH secretion in a number of ways including (a) inhibition of hormone synthesis, (b) inhibition of the enzyme converting pro-PTH to PTH, and (c) impairment of the release of hormone from the cell. Details of the control mechanisms and of the interactions between PTH calcitonin and vitamin D in calcium homeostasis will be considered in Chapter 12.

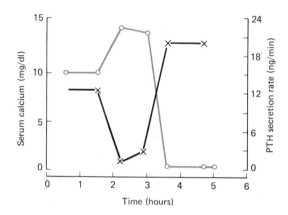

Figure 2.3 Changes in the secretion of PTH (x—x) from a goat's parathyroid gland resulting from changes in the concentration of calcium (o—o) in the perfusing blood, (Care, A. D., Sherwood, L. M., Potts, J. T. Jr. and Aurbach, G. D. Reprinted by permission from *Nature* **209**, 55. Copyright © 1966 Macmillan Journals Limited.)

Further reading

Daggett, Peter (1981). *Clinical Endocrinology*. Edward Arnold, London.
Greep, R. O. and Astwood, E. B. (1976). Endocrinology: Handbook of Physiology, Vol. VII. *Parathyroid Gland*. American Physiological Society, Washington.

3

The adrenal medulla

The adrenal medulla is functionally and embryologically part of the sympathetic nervous system. It secretes adrenaline (epinephrine) and noradrenaline (norepinephrine)—hormones which can influence the activity of virtually every tissue of the body.

Anatomy and microstructure

The adrenal glands are closely apposed to the rostral poles of the kidney: each is, in effect, two endocrine glands, the medulla, which secretes catecholamines, and the cortex (see Chapter 9), which secretes steroids. The polyhedral cells of the medulla are derived from neural crest material and can be considered as postganglionic sympathetic cells which have lost their axons and which release their secretions directly into the blood. They are supplied by preganglionic sympathetic nerve fibres which run from the lateral columns of the spinal grey matter to the gland via the splanchnic nerves.

The medullary cells are arranged in a series of irregular columns which closely invest the venous sinusoids. Each cell has within it prominent 'dense-cored vesicles' (chromaffin granules) which contain the catecholamines. There are strong indications from electron microscopic studies that there are two principal cell types within the medulla—'adrenaline-storing' cells and 'noradrenaline-storing' cells— within which the vesicles contain, virtually exclusively, the corresponding catecholamines. In adult man, adrenaline accounts for approximately 80 per cent of the stored medullary catecholamines, but in the fetus of all species and the newborn of many species there are few, if any, 'adrenaline-storing' cells. This is probably related to the functional maturation of the adrenal cortex, since glucocorticoids are known to be necessary for the induction of the enzyme which converts noradrenaline to adrenaline.

The adrenal medulla stains a deep yellow-brown with potassium dichromate—hence the term chromaffin. Chromaffin tissue is also found in retroperitoneal tissues, the mediastinum and occasionally in the neck. This extra-adrenal chromaffin tissue contains catecholamines: it is prominent in the fetus and newborn but undergoes progressive involution after birth: remnants of extra-adrenal chromaffin tissue may give rise to noradrenaline-secreting phaeochromocytomas in later life (see p.23).

Chemistry and metabolism of catecholamines

There are three important physiologically active catecholamines known so far (Fig. 3.1); of these *dopamine* is a neurotransmitter in the brain and a precursor of *noradrenaline*. Noradrenaline is released by postganglionic sympathetic nerve terminals, by certain cells in the brain, and by the adrenal medulla. *Adrenaline,* which is only released by the adrenal medulla, and possibly certain brain cells, is synthesized from noradrenaline.

The biosynthesis of the three principal catecholamines from the amino acid, phenylalanine, is illustrated in Fig. 3.1. Tyrosine, formed in the liver by hydroxylation of phenylalanine, is transported to postganglionic sympathetic nerve terminals or the adrenal medulla in the blood, from which it actively enters the cell. Once within the cells it is converted by tyrosine hydroxylase to dihydroxphenylalanine (DOPA) and thence to dopamine by the action of aromatic L-amino acid decarboxylase: both these reactions occur within the cytoplasm. The former reaction is probably rate-limiting to the entire synthetic sequence and, since tyrosine hydroxylase is inhibited by catecholamines, this serves to stabilize their synthesis and maintain optimal

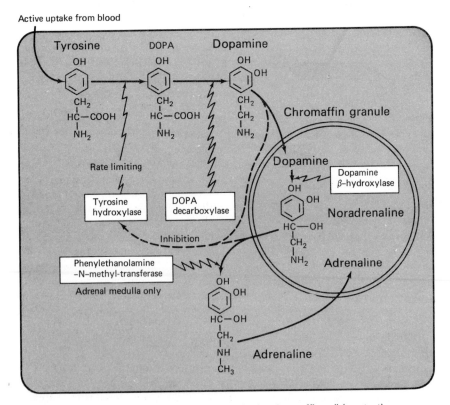

Figure 3.1 The synthesis of catecholamines within the chromaffin cell (see text). NB – – – indicates inhibition of tyrosine hydroxylase by dopamine and noradrenaline.

levels in the secretory cells. Dopamine enters the dense-core vesicles where it is converted by dopamine β-hydroxylase to noradrenaline. This is the end of the process in noradrenergic sympathetic nerve terminals and in the 'noradrenaline-storing' cells of the adrenal medulla, but, in the medullary 'adrenaline-storing' cells, noradrenaline passes from the vesicles into the cytoplasm once more. Here a final methylation occurs under the influence of phenylethanolamine-N-methyl-transferase producing adrenaline: this then migrates back into the vesicles prior to release from the cell.

The chromaffin granules act as a membrane-bound store principally for catecholamines, but they also contain the enzyme dopamine-β-hydroxylase, a remarkably high content of adenine nucleotides, particularly ATP, and a mysterious family of protein substances, called chromogranins, of unknown function.

The adrenal medulla is probably the only endocrine gland which has a true secretomotor innervation and, as such, can almost be considered analogous to an exocrine gland without ducts.

The mechanism which links the arrival of nerve impulses in the splanchnic nerves to the actual release of catecholamines into the blood is called **stimulus-secretion coupling** and has been the subject of extensive study. In essence, what is believed to happen is as follows.

1. Arrival of nerve impulses results in release of acetylcholine (ACh) from the nerve terminal.
2. The medullary cell membrane is depolarized by ACh.
3. As a result of (2), Ca^{2+} rapidly enters the cell.
4. Ca^{2+} in some way increases the probability that the membrane surrounding the chromaffin granules will fuse with the cell membrane.
5. The fused membranes break down allowing the vesicles to expel their contents into the extracellular space and hence the blood (exocytosis). (Ca^{2+} is probably involved in membrane breakdown and ATP may be implicated in the expulsion mechanism.)

Adrenaline and noradrenaline released from the adrenal medulla are physiologically inactivated extremely rapidly (Fig. 3.2). This may occur in one of two ways. Either the hormones are physically removed from the circulation by uptake into noradrenergic nerve terminals or other tissues, or they are broken down within the blood and tissues by catechol-O-methyl-transferase (COMT). Catechol-O-methyltransferase is widely distributed, but is particularly abundant in the brain, liver and kidneys. Adrenaline and noradrenaline are O-methylated by this enzyme forming metadrenaline and normetadrenaline respectively. These metabolites are largely excreted in the urine and thus measurement of urinary loss can provide a useful indication of catecholamine secretion. Alternatively, the O-methylated derivates may be oxidized ultimately to 3-methoxy-4-hydroxy-mandelic acid (vanillylmandelic acid, VMA). The reuptake of noradrenaline into sympathetic nerve terminals is probably quantitatively the most important means of removing this neuro-transmitter from its site of action, but such reuptake is also of considerable significance in removing catecholamines originating from the adrenal medulla. Following uptake into a nerve terminal, the amines may be

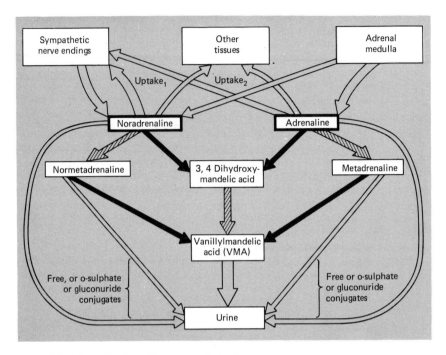

Figure 3.2 Metabolic disposition of catecholamines.
➡ steps controlled by monoamine oxidase (mAo). This enzyme is found chiefly in mitochondria, especially those in sympathetic nerve endings. It is also abundant in the liver and smooth muscle. It plays an important role in the disposal of catecholamines within nerve endings after reuptake or leakage from vesicles.
⟹ steps controlled by catechol-O-methyltransferase (COMT). This enzyme is confined largely to the soluble cytoplasmic compartment of sympathetic effector cells and the liver; there is little, if any, in sympathetic nerve endings. It is principally concerned with terminating the action of catecholamines after their release, either at the effector cell level or in the liver. *Note.* the width of the arrows gives a semi-quantitative index of the relative importance of the various metabolic pathways.

incorporated within a chromaffin granule or oxidized by mitochondrial or cytoplasmic monoamine oxidase (MAO). The uptake process appears to depend upon the presence of MAO, for, if the enzyme is inhibited, uptake is severely reduced as the chromaffin granules become replete.

The intraneural uptake of catecholamines has recently been designated uptake$_1$, for it has been found that catecholamines are also taken up by other tissues, such as smooth muscle: this process is called uptake$_2$. The significance of uptake$_2$ is still unclear, although the marked preference for adrenaline exhibited by extraneuronal tissues suggests that it may be of particular importance in removing and inactivating adrenaline secreted by the adrenal medulla.

Action of catecholamines on target tissues

The physiological actions of noradrenaline and adrenaline released into the blood from the adrenal medulla cannot be considered in isolation, because their release is invariably associated with activity in the sympathetic nervous system as a whole, and consequently with the release of noradrenaline from sympathetic nerve endings directly onto specific cells. Moreover, in almost all cases where quantitative studies have been attempted, it appears that circulating catecholamines of medullary origin are much less important than the direct neural stimulus.

In 1929, W. B. Cannon suggested that the sympathetic nervous system comprised an emergency mechanism brought into action under conditions of 'fright, fight or flight'—the so-called 'sympathetic discharge'. While it is certainly true that the sympathetic discharge is an essential component of the emergency response, the sympathetic nervous system plays a fundamental role in many homeostatic mechanisms under normal circumstances: the role of the adrenal medulla under the latter conditions is less well established.

Table 3.1 Adrenergic receptor classification

Tissue and effect		Receptor
Heart		
↑ Rate		β
↑ Contractility		β
Blood vessels		
Arterial constriction		α
Arterial dilation (muscle)		β
Venoconstriction		α
Other smooth muscle		
Bronchioles (dilation)		β
Spleen	(contraction)	α
	(relaxation)	β
Nictitating membrane	(contraction)	α
	(relaxation)	β
Iris radial muscle	(contraction)	α
Exocrine glands		
Pancreatic secretion		α
Salivary secretion		β
Sweat (apocrine)		α
Endocrine glands		
β cell: insulin (inhibition)		α
(stimulation)		β
α cell: glucagon (stimulation)		β
Metabolism		
Glycogenolysis		β
Lipolysis		β
Calorigenesis		β

Adrenergic receptors

The cellular effects of catecholamines follow the combination of the neurotransmitter or hormone with specific receptor sites on, or perhaps occasionally inside, the cells (adrenergic receptors). Ahlquist, in 1948, suggested that adrenergic receptors were of two types; α and β. Subsequently, there has been ample confirmation of this hypothesis both from measurements of the relative potency on particular tissues of adrenaline, noradrenaline and isoprenaline (a synthetic catecholamine) and as a result of studies of the specific inhibitory effects of drugs (α and β adrenergic blocking agents). As a first approximation, α receptors respond preferentially to noradrenaline and α actions generally involve the contraction of smooth muscle; β receptors respond principally to adrenaline and involve relaxation of smooth muscle or metabolic effects (see below). Furthermore, most β effects are brought about by the activation of adenyl cyclase, while many α effects are associated with inhibition of this enzyme. There are, of course, exceptions to the above generalizations, as will become clear from an examination of Table 3.1, which lists some of the types of adrenergic receptors found in specific tissues.

Cardiovascular effects
It is not within the scope of this book to discuss in detail the cardiovascular effects of catecholamines; however, they will be briefly summarized.

Adrenaline and noradrenaline increase heart rate through their action on the S–A node (chronotropic effect); they also increase myocardial contractility (inotropic effect) and may cause vasodilation of the coronary vessels. All these are β effects and serve potentially to augment the cardiac output. Vasoconstriction in all parts of the peripheral circulation can occur as a result of α activation by noradrenaline, usually of neural origin. However, adrenaline from the adrenal medulla mediates β adrenergic vasodilation in skeletal muscle.

Metabolic effects
The metabolic effects of catecholamines will be considered in detail in Chapter 11. Breakdown of hepatic glycogen (glycogenolysis), breakdown of fat stores (lipolysis) and increased heat production and oxygen consumption by many tissues (calorigenesis) are all β adrenergic effects. Insulin release is also inhibited by an α effect of catecholamines.

Other effects
Catecholamines have a number of actions on the alimentary tract and its secretions; they can also cause sweating, pilo-erection and bronchodilation (Table 3.1). Furthermore, they have a number of important effects on the central nervous system.

The sympathetic discharge
The concerted discharge of the sympathetic system and the associated stimulation of adrenomedullary secretion serve to produce in an animal a complex emergency response which, as Cannon realized, is well suited to

prepare it for fight or flight. Thus, the blood pressure and cardiac output increase and blood is diverted to skeletal muscle; glycogenolysis and lipolysis help provide substrate for muscle metabolism; bronchodilation and respiratory stimulation increase respiratory gas exchange; the spleen contracts and effectively transfuses erythrocyte-rich additional blood into the general circulation and pilo-erection helps to give subhuman species a more awe-inspiring appearance! It should be noted, however, that the sympathetic discharge is associated with the activation of other physiological responses, particularly stimulation of the pituitary-adrenocortical axis (Chapter 9).

Effects of deficiency

Unlike the adrenal cortex, the adrenal medulla does not appear to be essential to life. Thus demedullated animals survive well in the absence of severe stress, whereas, in most species, bilateral adrenalectomy results in death after a very short period. Presumably, the adrenal medulla is expendable because all its vital functions can be subsumed within the activity of the sympathetic nervous system. There is no recognized syndrome of adrenomedullary insufficiency in the clinical literature.

Effects of excess

Accidental massive overdose of either adrenaline or noradrenaline is lethal; it may cause fatal arrhythmias or a drastic increase in blood pressure which either induces cardiac failure or precipitates cerebral haemorrhage.

Chronic hypersecretion of catecholamines is encountered in patients with tumours of cells associated embryologically with the adrenal medulla.

> There are three major tumour types (all rare): the neuroblastoma derived from the primitive stem cell; the ganglioneuroma derived from the differentiated ganglion cell and phaeochromocytoma derived from the chromaffin cells. Neuroblastomas are highly malignant, ganglioneuromas are benign, and about 75 per cent of these two types of tumours secrete noradrenaline, they rarely secrete adrenaline. These tumours will not be considered further.
>
> Phaeochromocytomas are usually benign and may secrete exclusively noradrenaline, or more usually a mixture of adrenaline and noradrenaline (Daggett: *Clinical Endocrinology,* Chapter 5). In the latter case, this is taken to indicate that the cells have a medullary origin. The symptoms of phaeochromocytomas can be related to the relative properties of amines secreted and also to whether the secretion is continuous or episodic. In the former case, sustained hypertension results and in the majority of cases blood glucose is raised and the basal metabolic rate (BMR) elevated. If catecholamine secretion is intermittent, blood pressure may be normal or only slightly elevated while the tumour is quiescent. However, dramatic, but relatively transient increases in blood pressure (paroxysmal hypertension) result when the tumour becomes active: this may occur spontaneously or may be associated with emotion or exercise or with mechanical stimulation of the tumour during physical examination or surgical procedures. Paroxysmal hypertension is usually accompanied by hyper-glycaemia and may cause death from circulatory failure, cerebral haemorrhage or pulmonary oedema.

The condition can usually be temporarily alleviated by administration of an α blocking agent such as phentolamine: the fall in blood pressure seen in patients with catecholamine-producing tumours when given this drug is also of diagnostic value. The most effective form of treatment is surgical removal of the tumour.

Control of adrenomedullary secretion

Stimuli known to promote adrenomedullary secretion

The adrenal medulla probably has no resting secretion but can be provoked to release catecholamines in response to a variety of 'stressful' circumstances such as hypoxia, asphyxia, acidaemia, hypoglycaemia, hypothermia, hypotension, haemorrhage and exercise. Moreover, many emotional reactions, such as fear, anger, pain and sexual excitement, may be accompanied by adrenomedullary stimulation. With one exception, in all cases cited above the activity of the adrenal medulla is the result of stimulation via the splanchnic nerves. The exception is found in the fetus where it has been shown that the medulla is directly sensitive to hypoxia and asphyxia and will release noradrenaline before the splanchnic nerves have functionally developed. However, at the stage of development when the normal nervous link becomes effective, the direct medullary sensitivity to these stimuli effectively disappears. Indeed, thereafter the adrenal medulla becomes functionally inert if the splanchnic nerves are sectioned.

Assessment of adrenomedullary function

Ultrastructural studies indicate strongly that there are two types of chromaffin cell within the adrenal medulla; moreover, it is now well established that there are pronounced differences in the actions of the two amines on effector tissues. It would clearly be of considerable advantage to an animal to have independent nervous control of the secretion of each medullary hormone, and there have been many attempts to demonstrate differential control of the two groups of medullary cell.

There are, however, major technical problems associated with such studies, which merit consideration not only in the particular context of the adrenal medulla, but also in relation to experimental attempts to quantify the function of other endocrine glands.

Estimation of adrenomedullary secretion from blood concentration or urinary excretion of catecholamines
Some workers have attempted to evaluate adrenomedullary secretion in conscious animals and human subjects by measuring the concentrations of the two catecholamines in the blood (Daggett: *Clinical Endocrinology,* Chapter 5). At first sight, this may seem a not unreasonable approach; however, experience has shown it to be unsatisfactory for the following reasons.

1. The amount of any hormone in the plasma represents the algebraic sum of its rate of entry into blood from its site of production and its rate of loss due to peripheral utilization, breakdown or excretion. Consequently, unless the rate of

loss has been accurately measured, it is impossible to speculate usefully about its rate of production.

2. In the particular case of the medullary catecholamines, the problem is exacerbated by three further factors: first, the hormones are removed from the circulation very rapidly by a variety of methods (p.19); secondly, noradrenaline is produced in large quantities from the sympathetic nerve terminals and, finally, the plasma concentrations are too low to allow reliable estimation.

Attempts to quantify adrenomedullary secretion by extrapolation from estimations of the urinary loss of the catecholamines or their breakdown products provide at the most only crude semi-quantitative estimates, although this technique is a valuable clinical diagnostic procedure.

Collection of adrenal venous blood in anaesthetized animals
There have been many measurements of adrenomedullary catecholamine output in anaesthetized animals with a cannula placed in the adrenal vein. This method permits collection of the adrenal effluent blood, thus it is easy to compute the hormone output directly from measurements of arterial plasma concentration, adrenal venous plasma concentration and the blood flow. Unfortunately, this technique suffers from one insurmountable disadvantage—the animal is under an anaesthetic and has been subjected to extensive surgery. Both the adrenal medulla and the adrenal cortex are extremely sensitive to stress and there are few better ways of stressing an animal than anaesthesia and surgery! Furthermore, the anaesthetic will almost certainly affect those parts of the central nervous system concerned with adrenomedullary control. Consequently, although such techniques indubitably provide information about the responses of the adrenal medulla in anaesthetized animals, they contribute little to our understanding of the normal responses in the conscious animal.

Studies in conscious animals
There have been relatively few successful attempts to obtain adrenal venous blood from conscious animals with the gland *in situ*. Probably the most satisfactory method, and certainly the one which has found most application in the study of the selective secretion of catecholamines, is the 'adrenal clamp' technique (Fig. 3.3). During preliminary surgery the right kidney is removed from the young calves and a cannula is placed in the renal vein. A specially designed clamp is then inserted to divert adrenal venous blood into the root of the renal vein, where it travels round the clamp and returns to the vena cava. Application of a snare diverts adrenal blood from the return channel and allows collection from the renal vein cannula. After the operation, the collection tube and the snare control are left accessible outside the abdominal wall, thereby permitting collection of adrenal venous samples at will and without disturbance to the animal.

The results of the experiments using the 'adrenal clamp' technique have, as yet, provided no convincing evidence for a differential release of the two amines from the adrenal medulla in amounts which differ significantly from the storage ratio. Such stimuli as hypoglycaemia, hypoxia and hypercapnia all provide evidence for a predominant release of adrenaline. It remains to be seen whether this technique will reveal differences in the ratio of amines when the animal is exposed to other stimuli such as cold or haemorrhage.

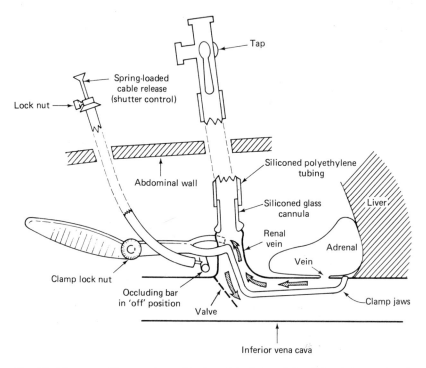

Fig. 3.3 Diagram to illustrate the positioning of the 'adrenal clamp' in relation to the adrenal gland and renal vein. (From Edwards, A. V., Hardy, R. N. and Malinowska, K.W. (1974). *Journal of Physiology* **239**, 477.)

4

The pancreatic islets

The pancreatic islets, or islets of Langerhans, are irregularly shaped, roughly ovoid clusters of endocrine cells which are scattered about between the acini in the pancreas. Removal of the gland results in death from **diabetes mellitus,** in the absence of appropriate treatment. This is because the β (B) cells of the islets represent the only effective source of the hormone **insulin,** which controls the rate at which glucose is delivered to peripheral tissues.

The α (A) cells of the pancreatic islets secrete **glucagon,** which also has important metabolic actions in the body that generally antagonize the effects of insulin. A third type of granular cell, the δ (D) cell, contains **somatostatin** (see p.74).

Results of recent studies using immunological techniques suggest the existence of pancreatic endocrine cells outside the islets altogether. In several species, including man, small clumps of cells situated between the acinar cells contain a peptide, comprising 36 amino acid residues, which has been called **pancreatic polypeptide** (PP). In man, there is a rapid rise in the concentration of this peptide in the blood after a meal, just as there is of insulin. In general, its actions appear to be reverse of those exerted by pancreozymin-cholecystokinin (CCK) (see Chapter 5); thus it inhibits the gallbladder and also the output of pancreatic enzymes. However, at this time PP can be regarded as no more than a putative hormone and it will not, therefore, be considered further here.

Anatomy and microstructure of gland

The pancreas develops from two diverticula that arise from the duodenum just behind the primordial liver. These develop into dorsal and ventral pancreases which then fuse and give rise to a single gland, but with two separate ducts. The gland develops in close association with the liver and the effluent blood drains directly into the portal vein. This fact may well have functional significance considering the importance of the actions both insulin and glucagon exert on the liver.

In the human fetus the endocrine cells develop, during the tenth to eleventh week, from small clusters of cells with dark cytoplasm which bud off from the developing ducts. Thus, by origin, the islets can be traced back to the duct epithelium, which is itself an outgrowth of duodenal endoderm, and they may therefore be regarded as endocrine specializations of the duodenal mucosa. No doubt the structural similarities between the molecules of certain pancreatic (glucagon) and intestinal hormones (enteroglucagon, secretin) reflect this common origin.

Insulin is detectable by the twelfth week in human fetal pancreas and granules are identifiable within the β cells a few days later. Thereafter the islets grow rapidly, and by four months account for roughly one-third of the total pancreatic mass. The knowledge that insulin production precedes that of the pancreatic enzymes was capitalized on by Banting and Best, who used simple saline extracts of fetal calf pancreas for many of their early experiments.

In the adult human pancreas there are between 200 000 and 1 800 000 islets, each about 75 × 175 nm, scattered between the acini, from which they are almost completely separated by a thin reticular membrane. The islet cells are arranged in irregular columns assembled around a labyrinth of anastomosing capillaries. The islets are highly vascular (a characteristic of endocrine tissue) and are also richly innervated by autonomic nerve terminals, which play an important part in controlling the release of both insulin and glucagon. The islet cells contain numerous granules which represent an intracellular store of hormone and are visible with the light microscope (Table 4.1). In most species, β cells predominate in the centre and α cells in the

Table 4.1   Common types of islet cell

Type	Proportion	Function	Characteristic feature
Alpha, α, A	20–30%	Glucagon secretion	Contain granules of uniformly high electron density
Beta, β, B	60–80%	Insulin secretion	Granules may have a characteristic crystalline appearance
Delta, δ, D	up to 8%	Contains somatostatin	Contain large granules of low electron density
PP	Variable*	Pancreatic polypeptide secretion	Contain granules of moderate to high electron density

*PP cells are also found in the exocrine part of the pancreas.

periphery of the islets. The D cells are usually scattered thinly between the two regions and, since somatostatin effectively inhibits release of both insulin and glucagon, it has been suggested that these cells exert some paracrine regulatory action on the rate at which the two hormones are released.

The physiology of insulin and glucagon will now be considered in turn, before returning to discuss the overall control of islet function.

Insulin

Chemistry and metabolism

Insulin is a small protein and was the first in which the amino acid sequence was mapped. It occurs in all vertebrate species and some invertebrates, and there are minor variations in the sequence of amino acids from species to species. However, the molecule invariably consists of two chains of amino acids which are joined together by three S–S bridges (necessarily, therefore, from cysteine to cysteine in each case; see Fig. 4.1 for structure of human insulin). These three disulphide linkages maintain the constant three-dimensional structure of the molecule first described by Dorothy Hodgkin in 1969.

The fact that insulin is a protein, and therefore potentially antigenic, provides a possible explanation for the fact that certain diabetic patients develop a resistance to insulins extracted from some species (particularly cattle and sheep) but respond normally to other insulin preparations (e.g. pig).

The hormone is derived from a single-chain precursor, called proinsulin, which is synthesized in the rough endoplasmic reticulum. The molecule has a spiral structure and a small amount may be released unchanged. Most is converted to insulin, however, in or near the Golgi apparatus, by tryptic cleavage, thus explaining the biosynthesis of the two-chain structure. The hormone is then stored in granular form until it is released by exocytosis in response to some specific stimulus. Glucose is thought to influence events both by promoting synthesis of proinsulin and by favouring Ca^{2+} entry, which activates the microtubule system thereby drawing granules to the surface of the cell and initiating secretion. Tryptic digestion of proinsulin produces two main products—insulin and the C (connecting) peptide, as illustrated in Fig. 4.2. The fact that release of insulin is accompanied by an equivalent molar amount of C peptide indicates that cleavage does not occur in the Golgi apparatus until after encapsulation of proinsulin. One is also left wondering whether this residual peptide fulfils some physiological function of which we are at present unaware.

Much of the insulin in the circulating plasma appears to be bound to a β-globulin, its half-life in the blood is short (about ten minutes) due to the avidity with which it is bound by various tissues, particularly liver and kidney; loss in the urine is small. In muscle and fat, insulin is broken down largely by proteolytic degradation, whereas in the liver enzymatic disruption of the disulphide linkage occurs due to the presence of **hepatic glutathione insulin transhydrogenase**.

In the past, this enzyme together with others which break down insulin, have been referred to collectively as 'insulinases' and it has been supposed that variations in the relative activities of 'insulinase' and 'insulinase-inhibitor' might explain such conditions as starvation diabetes. In fact, these enzymes appear to be nonspecific and are implicated in the degradation of a wide variety of hormones. Nor has any evidence emerged to support the view that variations in 'insulinase' and 'anti-insulinase' activity form a genuine homeostatic mechanism. It is known, however, that two separate proteins in the circulating plasma—an albumin and a $β_1$ lipoprotein—are capable of antagonizing the

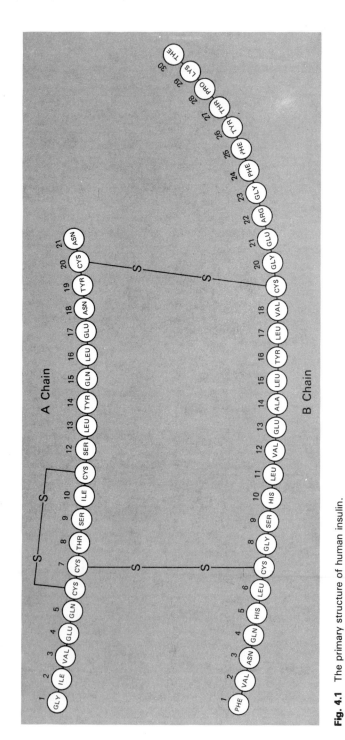

Fig. 4.1 The primary structure of human insulin.

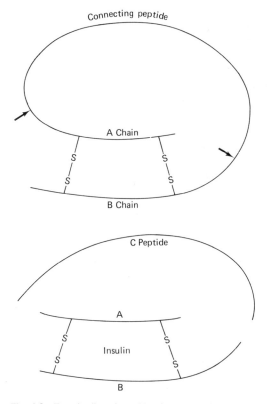

Fig. 4.2 Tryptic digestion of bovine or porcine proinsulin.

actions of insulin. The amounts of both can be increased in hypophysectomized animals by administration of growth hormone together with adrenal glucocorticoids, and abnormally high concentrations occur in diabetic patients.

Insulin was originally assayed by assessing its hypoglycaemic effect in the rabbit, but now insulin can be obtained in a pure, crystalline form and a reliable radio-immunoassay is available. The present International Standard defines the unit in terms of the weight of the hormone in crystalline form: 24.5 International Units = 1 mg zinc insulin.

When insulin is conjugated with other molecules (e.g. protamine or globin) it is possible to prolong the action of the hormone, and several such preparations are commercially available for the treatment of diabetes. However, since insulin is a protein and therefore rapidly digested in the gastrointestinal tract, they all have to be administered by injection.

Action of insulin on target tissues

Carbohydrate metabolism

The best known action of insulin is the way it lowers blood glucose concentration. This **hypoglycaemic** effect is a consequence both of an increased removal of glucose from the blood, following a facilitation of its uptake by certain tissues, and a decrease in glucose entry into the blood from glycogen stores in the liver.

Glucose uptake
Insulin is required for glucose entry into most cells, particularly muscle and adipose tissue which together comprise the major tissue mass in the body. In such 'insulin-sensitive' tissues the hormone affects the cell membrane by promoting a carrier-mediated transport system. Glucose is normally phosphorylated as soon as it enters the cell and so the internal concentration is very low. This means that net flux of glucose is virtually the same as glucose influx and therefore this is the rate-limiting step.. Hence the crucial importance of insulin in controlling the rate at which glucose is metabolized in most peripheral tissues.

Certain tissues do not require insulin for glucose entry. These include the CNS (except the satiety centre in the ventromedial hypothalamus), liver, intestinal epithelium, kidney tubular epithelium and the endocrine pancreas. (After you have read the section on diabetes consider how important each.of these exceptions is to an individual with an insulin deficiency.)

Effects on the liver
Insulin promotes the production of glycogen from glucose (glycogenesis) in the liver and muscle by induction of glycogen synthetase. It inhibits the breakdown of liver glycogen (glycogenolysis) (see Chapter 11) and also depresses the formation of glucose, from glucogenic amino acids such as alanine (gluconeogenesis).

Protein metabolism

Insulin promotes the transport of amino acids into liver and muscle cells. This process differs from the transport of glucose, in that amino acids are conveyed actively by expenditure of cellular energy against a concentration gradient. Transport of amino acids is linked to the Na^+/K^+ pump because binding of Na^+ to the carrier increases its affinity for amino acids.

Fat metabolism

Insulin inhibits the release of free fatty acids (FFA) and glycerol from fat depots (lipolysis), possibly by inhibiting adenyl cyclase in adipose tissue. Meanwhile, it promotes FFA synthesis from acetyl CoA in the liver at the expense of ketone body production

Glucagon secretion

There is some evidence that insulin may inhibit glucagon release from the α cells. In this connection, it is worth bearing in mind that the close proximity of β to α cells in the pancreatic islets may mean that the latter are exposed to higher concentrations of insulin than any other cell in the body, and that the α cells appear to be functionally linked to the β cells by 'gap' junctions.

Effects of insulin deficiency

As mentioned previously, *diabetes mellitus* is due to lack of insulin and varies in severity depending on the extent of the deficiency in insulin release. The disease occurs naturally in man and animals but the aetiology is still controversial.

Diabetes can be produced experimentally by any procedure which interferes with the production or release of insulin. As one would expect, removal of the pancreas results in severe diabetes which is rapidly fatal in the absence of replacement therapy. On the other hand, one can transplant the gland to some other part of the body without producing diabetes as long as an adequate blood supply is re-established. This shows that the islets are still capable of releasing sufficient insulin to prevent diabetes from occurring. However, it tells us nothing about the role of the innervation to the pancreatic islets under normal conditions.

Several chemicals selectively destroy the β cells and can be used to produce diabetes experimentally. By far the best known of these is alloxan, first discovered by Liebig in mucus from patients with dysentery. When injected in the right amount and under appropriate conditions, alloxan produces a very characteristic triphasic change in the blood glucose concentration. An initial moderate hyperglycaemia, due to cessation of insulin secretion, is followed by hypoglycaemia as the hormone is lost from the damaged β cells. Finally, the blood glucose concentration rises to the very high levels indicative of diabetes which persist unless the animal is given exogenous insulin. In newborn animals the hypoglycaemic phase is greatly exaggerated due to the large store of insulin which is present in the islets.

> Substances containing an $-SH$ group, such as glutathione, cysteine and dimercaprol, protect the β cell from the effects of alloxan if given immediately beforehand. This has led to the suggestion that alloxan acts by combining with $-SH$ groups, but it is worth noting that quite different substances, such as methylene blue, containing no $-SH$ groups, are also capable of protecting the β cell from alloxan. Over the years, alloxan has proved invaluable for producing selective β-cell destruction but it is a comparatively toxic substance and can cause damage to both the liver and kidneys. For this reason, most workers now prefer to use streptozotocin, which is an antibiotic and is less toxic to other tissues.

The consequences of insulin lack are shown diagrammatically in Fig. 4.3. Hyperglycaemia may be regarded as the primary defect and results both from an increased production of glucose in the liver and failure of peripheral tissues, such as muscle and fat, to take up glucose: 'starvation in the midst of plenty'. In the absence of insulin, the rate of glycogenolysis in the liver is enhanced and glycogenesis inhibited; gluconeogenesis is also favoured. The increased breakdown of fat leads to high levels of free fatty acids (FFA) in the plasma, which further inhibit the uptake of glucose by skeletal muscle and are metabolized to ketone bodies such as acetone, β-OH butyric and aceto-acetic acid in the liver (Daggett: *Clinical Endocrinology,* Chapter 2). The accumulation of these strong acids in the plasma leads to severe metabolic acidosis and the elimination of acetone in the lungs provides a useful diagnostic clue as it can readily be detected in the breath of ketotic diabetics. In skeletal muscle net

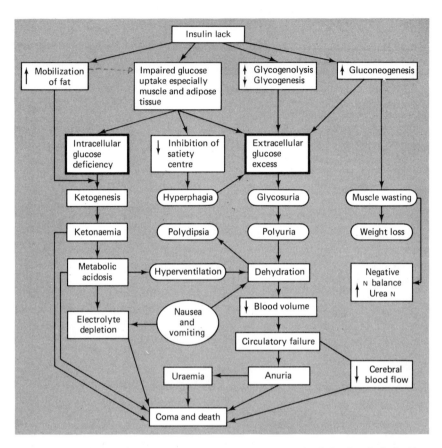

Fig. 4.3 Diagrammatic representation of the consequences of relative insulin lack. Note especially the principal pathways following a) 'Intracellular glucose deficiency' and b) 'Extracellular glucose excess'. Oval 'boxes' indicate the overt clinical features (see text).

protein catabolism becomes pronounced and the amino acids so produced provide further substrate for gluconeogenesis in the liver. This conversion of protein to glucose, which cannot be metabolized and is voided in the urine leads to rapid 'wasting' of the muscles, loss of weight and inanition in the untreated diabetic.

When the concentration of glucose in the plasma rises above the renal threshold (plasma glucose concentration of about 10 mmol/l or 180 mg/100 ml), the amount filtered at the glomerulus exceeds the capacity of the tubules to reabsorb it and glucose appears in the urine. The glucose that is not reabsorbed in the proximal convoluted tubule exerts a powerful osmotic effect and a profuse diuresis (polyuria) and associated thirst and drinking (polydipsia) are the most characteristic symptoms of the disease. Net loss of water and electrolytes in the kidney leads to pronounced dehydration and this is frequently exacerbated by further loss of fluid due to vomiting. Severe dehydration so reduces the blood volume as to cause circulatory failure and intense renal vasoconstriction. In the terminal stages, anuria leads to uraemia, coma and death.

The consequences of insulin lack described above can be regarded as acute in that they supervene within a matter of hours in the absence of insulin. In addition, there are long-term sequelae of the disease due to changes in arteries and capillaries. In general, healing is less efficient in diabetics and gangrene occurs much more commonly. Coronary, cerebral, renal and retinal arteries and arterioles are particularly prone to atherosclerotic changes and it has been found that the basement membranes of the capillaries are significantly thicker in diabetics than in non-diabetics.

Administration of insulin can correct most of the acute metabolic abnormalities which characterize the condition and allows diabetic patients to lead normal lives, except for the inconvenience of daily injections and the need to monitor their urine for the presence of glucose at frequent intervals. However, it is important to realize that it is a relative, rather than an absolute, lack of insulin which gives rise to diabetes. In 1936, Houssay showed that removal of the pituitary ameliorated the condition in dogs and that it was exacerbated by administration of pituitary extracts. In man, acromegaly (see Chapter 7) frequently causes diabetes. At about the same time, Long and Lukens demonstrated that the adrenal cortex also antagonizes insulin and that adrenalectomy leads to partial recovery from diabetes in pancreatectomized dogs. Furthermore, a proportion of diabetic patients are rather resistant to insulin and require very high doses of the hormone. Thus, in theory, hyperactivity of anti-insulin mechanisms *could* give rise to the disease; in practice this happens comparatively rarely and resistance to insulin is often due to the presence of insulin antibodies which interfere with its biological activity.

Diabetes first becomes apparent either during childhood (juvenile diabetes) or in later life, after the age of forty (maturity-onset diabetes) (Daggett: *Clinical Endocrinology,* Chapter 2). In juvenile diabetics virtually all the β cells in the pancreas may be absent or damaged and regular injections of insulin are the only satisfactory treatment. When diabetes appears later in life it is frequently associated with obesity and can often be controlled merely by dieting. Alternatively, injections of insulin may be avoided by the use of some oral hypoglycaemic agent, such as tolbutamide. This drug acts by stimulating the release of endogenous insulin and is therefore only effective in patients in whom there is some persistent β-cell function.

Effects of insulin excess

Excessive production of endogenous insulin is often referred to as 'inappropriate insulin release', because it is inappropriate to metabolic requirement. However, the effects of excess insulin are most commonly encountered in insulin-dependent diabetics and result from overdose (Daggett: *Clinical Endocrinology,* Chapter 2).

Very rarely, this occurs as a side-effect of neoplasia. In adults, primary insulin-secreting tumours of the pancreas (insulinomas) may develop and a diffuse proliferation of β-cell precursors (nesidioblasts) has been described in babies. This condition has been given the name nesidioblastosis and causes chronic hypoglycaemia due to hyperinsulinism. The comparative inefficiency of the insulin-release mechanism in the neonate has been well documented but it is worth noting here that hypoglycaemia may occur in babies who have been given glucose by intravenous infusion, shortly after the infusion is discontinued. This seems to be due to persistent release of insulin after removal of the hyperglycaemic stimulus and shows that the islets are slow to respond both to onset and offset of stimulation for some time after birth. The point is worth stressing because it provides a partial explanation for the hypoglycaemia which can occur immediately after birth in the babies of diabetic mothers. In this situation, the fetus continually receives much more glucose than it requires by facilitated transfer across the placenta. The fetal pancreas responds to this stimulus very efficiently by hypertrophy of islet tissue and increased insulin production, but when the placental supply of glucose is suddenly terminated at birth, the islets are slow to recognize this change in circumstances and continue to secrete rather large amounts of insulin.

Normally, the rate at which insulin is released from the pancreatic islets is modified by a wide range of different factors (see below) which together ensure that the requirements of the peripheral tissues for glucose are subservient to that of the brain. Daily or twice-daily injections of insulin, upon which many diabetics depend, are a clumsy alternative to the sophisticated mechanism by which insulin release is controlled naturally. Furthermore, the requirement for insulin can change abruptly in response to stress, mild disease, undue exercise and many other factors.

The effects of hyperinsulinism are entirely due to hypoglycaemia and the consequential failure of central nervous function.

Slices of brain *in vitro* are capable of metabolizing a wide variety of substrates (e.g. glucose, fructose, lactate, pyruvate, α-ketoglutarate, oxaloacetate) just like other tissues, but glucose is the only one which is transported across the blood–brain barrier sufficiently rapidly to provide an effective source of energy in the normal animal or man. This is why the respiratory quotient (RQ) of the brain is 1.0—that for glucose metabolism. If the central nervous system is provided with insufficient glucose, the small store of glycogen in the brain is very quickly exhausted and the RQ then falls as the neurones begin to break down other substances.

Although there is considerable variation in the signs of hypoglycaemia between individuals, the symptoms generally appear in a definite sequence and those that are most commonly observed are listed in Table 4.2. The pattern is dictated by the fact that, in both man and animals, the most highly specialized neurones are most sensitive to glucose deprivation and so cerebral function is disrupted long before the lower centres are affected. Sufficiently intense hypoglycaemia produces a form of rigidity which closely resembles that produced surgically in animals by decerebration. This disappears with persistent severe hypoglycaemia as the cells of the reticular formation eventually succumb in their turn.

Insulin-dependent diabetics should know that they are liable to

Table 4.2   Some of the more common symptoms and signs of hypoglycaemia in approximate sequence

1.	Confusion
2.	Yawning, lethargy, dizziness
3.	Signs of increased sympathetic activity
	Tachycardia
	Sweating together with cutaneous vasoconstriction producing a cold clammy skin
	Anxiety
4.	Collapse, convulsions
5.	Coma, decerebrate rigidity
6.	Respiratory paralysis → death

hypoglycaemic episodes consequent upon inadvertent overdosage, and that they only need to take one or two glucose tablets to raise their blood glucose concentration and avert the hazard. Fortunately, although the cerebral cortex is affected first, causing confusion, they are usually able to recognize what is happening to them and to take the necessary avoiding action. When glucose is administered, all the signs of hypoglycaemia disappear within minutes, unless the condition has been sufficiently severe and prolonged to produce neuronal damage.

Newborn babies differ from adults by being extremely resistant to hypoglycaemia and may not show any sign of abnormality with blood glucose concentrations below 20 mg/100 ml for hour after hour. This characteristic is shared by the newborn calf, in which the phenomenon has been investigated in some detail. Experiments in calves show that, during the first few days after birth, the brain is protected from the effects of intense hypoglycaemia by the release of adrenaline from the adrenal medulla. This causes a pronounced increase in blood lactate concentration due to glycogenolysis in skeletal muscle, and it seems likely that the brain can utilize this metabolite, in the absence of glucose, because the blood – brain barrier is more permeable to lactate at this stage of development. Adrenaline probably mobilizes other metabolites, such as free fatty acids and glycerol, which can cross the blood – brain barrier more easily in the newborn animal. It may also increase cerebral blood flow, thereby producing an increase in the supply of nutrients to the brain relative to other tissues.

Later in life, any lactic acid produced by mobilization of muscle glycogen is rapidly converted to glucose in the liver and then lost to the peripheral tissues because of the insulin excess. Thus the newborn animal is endowed with a special adrenergic mechanism which maintains cerebral metabolism in the absence of glucose. It operates for a limited period, during which the newborn animal is especially susceptible to hypoglycaemia because (a) it has to establish a gastrointestinal route for absorption of nutrients in place of placental transfer, and (b) the homeostatic mechanisms which maintain the blood glucose concentration in the adult are poorly developed.

In the adult, prolonged fasting leads to adaptive changes which enable the brain to utilize free fatty acids and ketone bodies in place of glucose. In any other circumstance, failure of the glucose supply to the brain results in death

Table 4.3 Mechanisms known to antagonize the effects of insulin during intense hypoglycaemia

Sensor	Mediator	Effector	Action
Hypothalamic centres	Sympathetic innervation to liver and	? Noradrenaline	Hepatic glycogenolysis
	adipose tissue	Noradrenaline	Lipolysis, ↑ FFA
Hypothalamic centres	Sympathetic innervation to adrenal medulla	Adrenaline	1. Hepatic glycogenolysis 2. Lipolysis, ↑ FFA
Hypothalamic centres	Sympathetic innervation to pancreas	? Noradrenaline	↓ Insulin release ↑ Glucagon release
Hypothalamic glucoreceptors	CRF/ACTH	Cortisol/ corticosterone	1. Lipolysis, ↑ FFA 2. Gluconeogenesis
α cells directly	Ca²⁺		Hepatic glycogenolysis
Hypothalamic glucoreceptors	Parasympathetic innervation to pancreatic islets	Glucagon	Gluconeogenesis
Hypothalamic centres	Sympathetic innervation to pancreatic islets		Lipolysis
Hypothalamic glucoreceptors	GHRF	Growth hormone	1. Antagonizes effect of insulin on glucose transport 2. Lipolysis, ↑ FFA

CRF = corticotrophin-releasing factor (p. 73); ACTH = adrenocorticotrophic hormone (corticotrophin) (p. 78); GHRF = growth hormone-releasing factor (p. 74); FFA = free fatty acids.

within a few hours and the importance of maintaining a normal blood glucose concentration is reflected in the number and variety of anti-insulin mechanisms which are activated during intense hypoglycaemia (Table 4.3).

The sympathetic system alone is capable of antagonizing excess insulin in at least four ways: direct stimulation of hepatic glycogenolysis, release of adrenaline from the adrenal medullae and glucagon from the pancreatic islets and inhibition of endogenous insulin release. However, the sympathetic system itself is relatively insensitive to the specific stimulus of hypoglycaemia and is probably more concerned with providing additional glucose during exercise than with glucose homeostasis. The hormonal mechanism which responds to hypoglycaemia most readily is undoubtedly the release of adrenal glucocorticoids, but it is still not entirely clear what acute effects they have that would tend to antagonize insulin. They are known to potentiate various adrenergic actions and it is possible that some such 'permissive' role is important under these conditions. Glucagon release (mediated by the parasympathetic innervation to the pancreatic islets) and growth-hormone release occur in response to moderate hypoglycaemia, but all the available evidence shows that the adrenal medulla is extremely resistant to hypoglycaemia.

Glucagon

Chemistry and metabolism

Pancreatic glucagon is a polypeptide hormone consisting of a single chain of 29 amino acids, with a molecular weight of 3485 (see Fig. 4.4).

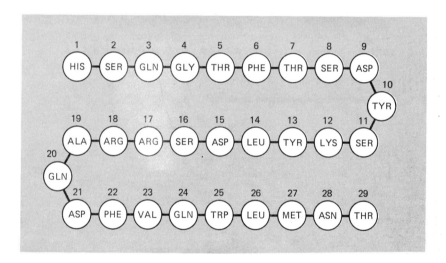

Fig. 4.4 Structures of porcine and bovine glucagon.

Pancreatic glucagon is synthesized and released from the α cells in the islets. These cells contain quite typical electron-dense secretory granules which are formed in the Golgi apparatus, become arranged in chains and migrate to the cell surface where they are released by exocytosis, as is insulin.

Very similar cells have been demonstrated in the gastrointestinal mucosa and represent the source of a similar hormone, which has been called enteroglucagon or, since it is measured by immunoassay, glucagon-like immunoreactivity of ileal origin. In spite of the fact that enteroglucagon resembles glucagon immunologically, it is a much larger molecule and has been found to be released in response to quite different stimuli. It must, therefore, be regarded as a separate entity. In the dog, but not in other species as far as we know, cells indistinguishable from pancreatic α cells occur in large numbers in the fundus of the stomach. These cells release a hormone which appears to be identical immunologically with pancreatic glucagon. It is also released in response to the same stimuli and produces the same peripheral effects as the pancreatic hormone.

The half-life of glucagon in the circulating plasma (approximately six minutes) is similar to that of insulin. Ten to fifteen minutes after an intravenous injection, the apparent distribution space is equal to the body volume, showing that there must have been substantial degradation as well as distribution of hormone. The rapidity with which glucagon disappears from the blood shows that it cannot be bound to plasma protein effectively and that it is taken up quickly by peripheral tissues. The hormone is rapidly degraded in plasma and samples of blood for glucagon assay therefore have to be treated with aprotonin, a kallikrein inhibitor, to prevent this occurring.

Glucagon is avidly taken up by the liver, in which it is bound to receptor sites and also rapidly degraded. Material immunologically resembling glucagon is also excreted in the bile. Substantial amounts of glucagon are degraded in the kidney, although virtually none is voided in the urine. It seems that the hormone is filtered through the glomeruli but then reabsorbed in the proximal convoluted tubule where it is also metabolized.

Action of glucagon on target tissues

It has been established that glucagon is capable of producing the following actions.

1. Glycogenolysis in the liver.
2. Inhibition of glycogen synthesis in the liver.
3. Gluconeogenesis in the liver.
4. Lipolysis in adipose tissue.
5. Stimulation of insulin release from β cells.
6. Stimulation of catecholamine release.
7. A positive inotropic effect on the heart.

Glucagon is the most powerful known hyperglycaemic agent: release of pancreatic glucagon in response to hypoglycaemia rapidly tends to restore the blood glucose concentration by mobilizing liver glycogen. It also acts more slowly to maintain the blood glucose concentration by promoting gluconeogenesis in the liver. The discovery that glucagon acts on the hepatocyte by activating adenyl cyclase and increasing the intracellular concentration of cAMP led to the formulation of the 'second messenger' concept by Earl Sutherland and his colleagues; it is now known that cAMP mediates the actions of more than half the hormones in the body (see p.000 and Table 1.3). Figure 4.5 illustrates the main steps that are thought to be involved in the stimulation of glycogenolysis in the liver. For ease of description, the steps are identified numerically in the flow diagram. Glucagon binds on the external surface of the hepatocyte (1) to highly specific receptors, of which there is a vast excess over the number which, when occupied, will produce a maximal rate of glycogenolysis (approximately 1 per cent). This large excess of receptor sites will have the effect of greatly

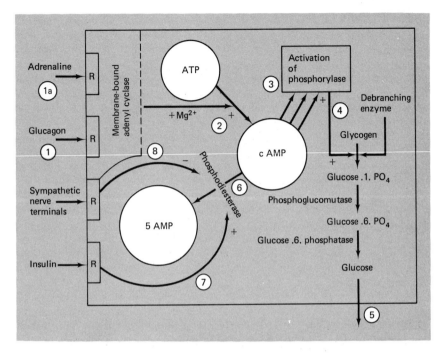

Fig. 4.5 A diagrammatic representation of the factors affecting glycogenolysis in a liver cell (see text for details).

increasing the sensitivity of the liver cell to the circulating hormone. Adrenaline also binds to receptors on the surface of the cell (1a) but they are quite different receptors and this action of adrenaline can be blocked by adrenergic blocking agents, whereas the glycogenolytic response to glucagon persists. Both glucagon and adrenaline, when bound to their respective receptors, activate membrane-bound adenyl cyclase which catalyses the conversion of ATP to $3'5'$ cAMP (2) in the presence of Mg^{2+}. However, comparison of the changes in cAMP concentration in response to these two hormones shows that glucagon is by far the more effective stimulus *in vitro*. *In vivo*, glucagon is released much more readily than adrenaline and is secreted directly into the portal blood, which passes immediately to the liver, so that glucagon plays a much more important role than adrenaline in control of hepatic glycogenolysis.

Cyclic AMP activates phosphorylase in the liver (3) by stepwise activation, first of a protein kinase, then phosphorylase kinase and finally phosphorylase itself by splitting off a PO_4 group from the enzyme. Phosphorylase, together with the debranching enzyme, catalyses the conversion of glycogen to glucose.1.PO_4 (4) and thence, via glucose.6.PO_4 to free glucose which passes out of the cell down its concentration gradient (5). The effect of this cascade of enzyme reactions is to magnify the effect of the hormone to such an extent that the attachment of a single molecule of glucagon to its specific receptor results in the production of about 3 000 000 molecules of glucose.

Cyclic AMP itself is broken down to 5AMP in the presence of phosphodiesterase, and two quite separate control mechanisms are now known to influence the rate at which glycogen is converted into glucose in the liver by controlling the rate of degradation of this enzyme. First, insulin acts by increasing the concentration of phosphodiesterase (7) thereby reducing the intracellular concentration of cAMP and thus inhibiting the rate of glycogenolysis. These cells are also extremely sensitive to stimulation via the sympathetic innervation and the response is not blocked by adrenergic blocking agents. It therefore appears that stimulation of these nerve terminals leads to the activation of different receptors; the effect is then to inhibit phosphodiesterase and thereby increase the cAMP concentration so promoting glycogenolysis (8). (Methyl xanthines, such as aminophylline, also inhibit phosphodiesterase and are used experimentally to raise the intracellular concentration of cAMP). As noted in the listed actions of insulin, this hormone actively promotes glycogenesis by induction of glycogen synthetase. Recent studies show that this enzyme is also induced in response to stimulation of the parasympathetic innervation to the liver, providing yet another example of antagonism between the two divisions of the autonomic nervous system.

In addition to producing a rapid rise in blood glucose concentration by promoting the breakdown of liver glycogen, glucagon acts more slowly to make glucose available from protein by gluconeogenesis. It also has a pronounced lipolytic effect and the free fatty acids produced are metabolized preferentially by muscle, thereby conserving glucose for cerebral use. The physiological significance of the other actions of glucagon listed above (stimulation of insulin release, stimulation of catecholamine release, positive inotropic effect) have not yet been established and they will not, therefore, be considered further here.

Effects of glucagon deficiency

No clinical condition attributable specifically to lack of glucagon has yet been described. However, it seems likely that growth hormone exerts a trophic action on the pancreatic α cells and that glucagon release is impaired in cases of panhypopituitarism. The metabolic consequences of this deficit, if any, have not been elucidated.

Effects of glucagon excess

Most forms of stress have been shown to cause hyperglucagonaemia. In many cases the release of pancreatic glucagon is probably mediated by the sympathetic innervation to the islets, but the α cells are capable of responding directly to certain stresses, such as intense hypoxia. Thus, the release of glucagon and the consequent hyperglycaemia in response to hypoxia are not impaired by blocking the autonomic nerves to the α cell: glucagon-secreting tumours of the pancreas (glucagonomas) have also been described, but they are very rare (Daggett: *Clinical Endocrinology,* Chapter 3). The patients are mildly diabetic.

Far more important is the finding that the α cells are comparatively insensitive to glucose in diabetes mellitus. The plasma glucagon level is usually found to be within the normal range in untreated diabetics, even though the level of glucose is well above normal. In addition, the rise in plasma glucagon concentration in response to leucine (see p.44) is usually exaggerated in juvenile diabetics in spite of the hyperglycaemia. However, both the reduced sensitivity of the α cell to glucose and the enhanced response to leucine are restored towards normal by infusing small doses of insulin. It is therefore reasonable to conclude that defective α-cell function in diabetics is due, at least in part, to lack of insulin.

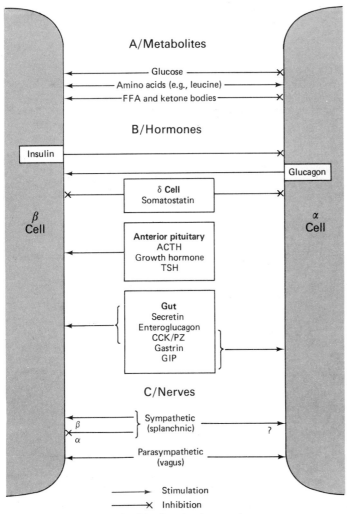

Fig. 4.6 Factors influencing islet function (see text).

The control of islet function

The control of glucagon and insulin secretion is complex and seemingly innumerable factors have been shown to influence the rates at which these two hormones are released. Cyclic nucleotides are intimately concerned in both release mechanisms, as are cations such as Na^+ and Ca^{2+} added to which various pharmacological agents are known to stimulate (e.g. tolbutamide) or inhibit (e.g. alloxan) islet-cell function. The following account is restricted to those metabolic, neural or hormonal factors which may play a part in controlling the release of glucagon or insulin from the pancreas under normal physiological conditions. (Fig. 4.6).

Metabolites

Glucose

Plasma glucose concentration is undoubtedly the most important of the factors which normally control the release of these hormones, stimulating release of insulin and inhibiting that of glucagon. Both the α and β cells are directly sensitive to the concentration of glucose in the surrounding fluid, but glucose is also monitored in the hypothalamus, which is probably even more sensitive to small fluctuations in concentration, and influences the rates of insulin and glucagon release via the autonomic innervation to the islets. The fact that the β cells are directly sensitive to glucose *in vivo* was first shown in conscious dogs with indwelling catheters in the pancreatico-duodenal artery. Local infusion of glucose into the pancreatic vascular bed over a period of two or three weeks was found to cause peripheral hypoglycaemia and, at post-mortem, the islets were found to be hypertrophied.

An interesting feature of islet function is the pronounced lability of the cell. Thus, starvation rapidly impairs release of insulin in response to glucose (within twenty-four hours) and the normal response is restored quite quickly by feeding. This is now thought to be due to changes in some glucose-inducible enzyme system in the β cell.

Amino acids

A wide range of amino acids, especially leucine, is known to stimulate release of both glucagon and insulin. Furthermore, there is considerable interaction between the effects exerted by the amino acids and that of glucose. Thus, insulin release in response to a protein meal is markedly potentiated by hyperglycaemia, while release of glucagon is effectively suppressed under the same conditions.

Free fatty acids, ketone bodies and volatile fatty acids

Free fatty acids and ketone bodies have a weak stimulatory effect on the β cell and tend to suppress α-cell activity, but it has yet to be proved that these effects are of any physiological significance. It is more likely that free fatty acids influence the islets by potentiating release of insulin in response to glucose. In ruminants, such as the sheep, in which all the carbohydrate in the diet is absorbed in the form of volatile fatty acids (acetate, propionate and butyrate), butyrate has been shown to stimulate release of insulin.

Hormones

Trophic effects

Normal growth and development of the pancreatic islets is critically dependent upon the hormonal climate. Several different hormones seem to be important in this respect, including growth hormone, thyroxine and the glucocorticoids, and in each case there is an optimum range which favours islet growth, above or below which development is impaired.

Glucagon and insulin

Both glucagon and insulin can be shown to influence the rate of secretion of the other. Insulin inhibits release of glucagon while glucagon stimulates secretion of insulin. The significance of these findings is still not entirely clear, but provides additional evidence in support of the view that the islets respond as a bihormonal unit under most circumstances and that it is the change in the insulin–glucagon ratio that is important in directing metabolism (see below).

Gastrointestinal hormones

Comparison of the tolerance to glucose administered intravenously or by intrajejunal infusion has shown that far higher blood glucose levels are achieved following administration by the intravenous route. This appears to be due to release of several gastrointestinal hormones which either stimulate release of insulin or potentiate release in response to glucose when it is administered via the gastrointestinal tract (Daggett: *Clinical Endocrinology,* Chapter 3). It is not known precisely which hormones promote insulin release during digestion, but secretin, pancreozymin/cholecystokinin (CCK/PZ) neurotensin and enteroglucagon are all likely candidates. In addition, gastrin, CCK/PZ and gastric-inhibitory peptide (GIP) can stimulate glucagon secretion under certain circumstances and may exert an important effect on the pancreatic islets during digestion and absorption.

Neural effects

Sympathetic system

It is now known that the pancreatic islets are extremely sensitive to stimulation via the sympathetic innervation. Secretion of glucagon is stimulated and insulin release is suppressed at stimulus frequencies well within the physiological range. The inhibitory effect on the β cell is mediated by α-adrenergic receptors and a β-adrenergic stimulatory effect is unmasked by α-blocking agents. However, the sympathetic system is rather insensitive to fluctuations in plasma glucose concentration and probably plays little part in maintaining plasma glucose concentration under normal conditions. It is probably far more important in modifying metabolism during exercise or stress.

Parasympathetic system

Even more recently, it has been shown that section of the vagus nerve or administration of atropine substantially reduces both the release of glucagon during moderate hypoglycaemia and the release of insulin which occurs when small amounts of glucose are infused intra-arterially to the brain. These parasympathetic mechanisms appear to be sufficiently sensitive to changes in plasma glucose concentration to participate in glucose homeostasis.

Coordinated islet responses

Insulin conserves metabolites by promoting glycogenesis, lipogenesis and protein synthesis when glucose and amino acids are plentiful, whereas glucagon ensures a sufficiency of glucose for cerebral metabolism at other times by promoting glycogenolysis, lipolysis and gluconeogenesis. The activities of the α and β cells appear coordinated to ensure that the glucagon:insulin ratio is appropriately adjusted. It is more important to understand how the islets respond in certain defined circumstances than to attempt to remember precisely how one particular stimulus affects one or other hormone.

Three common conditions are used as examples here and the ways in which glucose distribution is modified in response to a change in the glucagon:insulin ratio are represented diagrammatically in Fig. 4.7.

The resting postabsorptive state

Under normal resting conditions, small amounts of both glucagon and insulin are released and the input to the glucose pool from the liver precisely matches the uptake by the brain and peripheral tissues (Fig. 4.7a).

Exercise

During exercise, release of pancreatic glucagon rises abruptly while that of insulin is suppressed. Both effects are probably mediated via the sympathetic innervation to the islets. The net result of the rise in the glucagon:insulin ratio is a substantial increase in the output of glucose by the liver and of uptake by skeletal muscle, while the concentration of glucose in the plasma and the supply to the brain remains constant (Fig. 4.7b). Supportive effects of glucagon in this situation would include gluconeogenesis and mobilization of FFA by lipolysis.

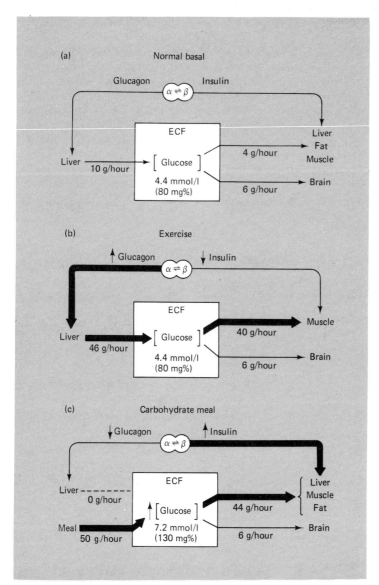

Fig. 4.7 A diagrammatic representation of the patterns of glucagon and insulin release at rest (**A**), during exercise (**B**) and following a meal of carbohydrate (**C**) and the consequential changes in glucagon distribution. (From Unger, R. H. (1976) Diabetes **25,** 136.)

The postprandial state

During absorption of nutrients following a meal consisting mainly of carbohydrates (such as students are frequently served), alimentary hyperglycaemia occurs. The rise in plasma glucose concentration, together with various humoral factors released from the gut, inhibit glucagon and strongly stimulate insulin release. The brain continues to take up the requisite amount of glucose; the excess pours into the peripheral tissues and is converted to glycogen in the liver and in muscle and to fat in adipose tissue (Fig. 4.7c).

Following a more expensive meal, consisting mainly of protein, the amino acids which are absorbed stimulate release of both glucagon and insulin. Insulin favours protein synthesis and glucagon ensures that hypoglycaemia is averted. The way in which insulin and glucagon are integrated into the overall endocrine regulation of energy metabolism will be discussed further in Chapter 11.

Further reading

Baba, S., Saki, H. and Imapura, Y. (Eds.) (1979). *Proinsulin, insulin, C-peptide.* Excerpta Medica, Amsterdam, Oxford.

Daggett, Peter (1981). *Clinical Endocrinology.* Edward Arnold, London.

Foa, P. P. and Bajaj, J. S. (Eds.) (1978). *Glucagon: its role in physiology and clinical medicine.* Springer-Verlag, New York.

Greep, R. O. and Astwood, E. B. (1972). Endocrinology: Handbook of Physiology, Vol. 1. *Endocrine Pancreas.* American Physiological Society, Washington.

Unger, R. H., Dobbs, R. E. and Orci, L. (1970). Insulin, glucagon, and somatostatin secretion in the regulation of metabolism. *Annual Review of Physiology* **40**, 307.

Unger, R. H. and Orci, L. (1976). Physiology and pathophysiology of glucagon. *Physiology Reviews* **56**, 778.

Vallance-Owen, J. (Ed.) (1975). *Diabetes.* MTP Press, Lancaster.

5

The gastrointestinal tract

The gastrointestinal mucosa is the largest and most diverse endocrine gland in the body (Daggett: *Clinical Endocrinology,* Chapter 3). It contains a great variety of cell types, many of which may have an endocrine function. However, these endocrine cells are not grouped together as is the case in almost all other hormone-secreting tissues, but are scattered as single cells amongst the other mucosal elements. This, coupled with the fact that the control of gastrointestinal secretion and motility is the result of a complex interaction of endocrine and autonomic nervous activity, makes the investigation of individual gastrointestinal hormones extremely difficult. One further complication is the strong possibility of **paracrine** activity see p.1, in which cells secrete specific chemicals which affect adjacent cells directly by diffusion rather than via the circulation. Such actions are of course extremely difficult to demonstrate experimentally *in vivo*.

A detailed consideration of the endocrine function of the alimentary canal lies beyond the scope of this book. Consequently, mention will be made of the characteristics of the few hormones generally recognized to be of physiological importance and a brief mention will be made of other, recently discovered, intestinal peptides which *may* be shown in the future to play a role in normal gut function.

Chemistry of gastrointestinal hormones and similar mucosal peptides

Gastrin

This hormone occurs in two main forms: 'gastrin 17' secreted from the pyloric antrum and 'gastrin 34' (big gastrin) secreted mainly from the upper small intestine. 'Gastrin 17' contains 17 amino acids with the C-terminal sequence:

$$Gly - Trp - Met - Asp - Phe \ (NH_2)$$

Big gastrin contains 34 amino acids, but includes the identical 17 to 'gastrin 17' at the C-terminal end. The half-life of G34 in plasma is about six times that of G17; consequently its action is more prolonged. Gastrin 34 is, in fact, about six times less effective in its actions than G17 so, on balance, they are practically equipotent.

Pancreozymin-cholecystokinin (CCK)

Pancreozymin-cholecystokinin is secreted by the duodenal mucosa and contains 33 amino acids, of which the C-terminal pentapeptide sequence is identical to that of gastrin (see above). In consequence, the actions of gastrin and CCK overlap and it has been shown that the C-terminal pentapeptide possesses the biological actions common to both hormones. The N-terminal sequences are responsible for the selectivity toward stimulation of acid secretion of gastrin and the pancreatic-enzyme stimulation and gallbladder-contracting effects of CCK.

Secretin

Secretin is released from certain cells in the mucosa of the duodenum and upper jejunum. It contains 27 amino acids and its structure is quite distinct from that of gastrin and CCK, but resembles in some respects that of glucagon, GIP and VIP (q.v.). Its particular claim to fame is, of course, the fact that it was the first hormone to be demonstrated (Bayliss and Starling, 1902). Ironically perhaps, some recent evidence has failed to show any rise in its secretion under physiological circumstances and consequently there are now doubts as to whether it really is a hormone!

Gastric inhibitory peptide (GIP)

Gastric inhibiting peptide is secreted from the duodenum, jejunum and upper ileum and contains 43 amino acids. Its structure resembles that of both secretin and glucagon.

Enteroglucagon

Enteroglucagon is found in the lower small intestine and colon in man. Its structure has not been elucidated, but, from immunological evidence, is probably similar to that of pancreatic glucagon (p.39): the plasma concentration has been shown to increase to a small extent some time after a meal.

The five peptide types mentioned above are, with the possible exception of secretin, considered by most authorities to be hormones, to the extent that they are secreted in response to specific stimuli and manifest defined effects on target cells when present in the blood at physiological concentrations. Some of these actions are listed in Table 5.1 and an impression of the potential complexity of their interactions may be obtained from Fig. 5.1, which is *not* intended to be committed to memory! (The notation of particular actions, G1, G2, etc. in Table 5.1, corresponds with that in Fig. 5.1). Endocrine effects on

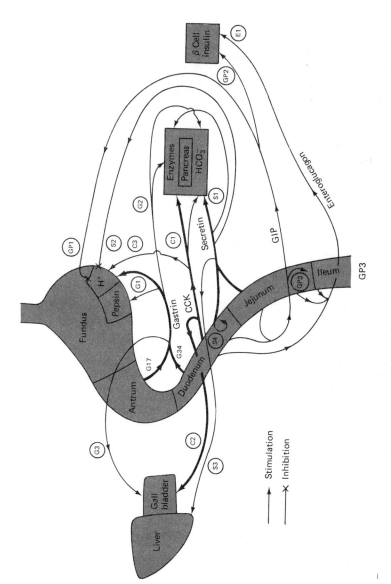

Fig. 5.1 Diagram to show the source and principal actions of gastrin, CCK, secretin, GIP and enteroglucagon. Notation (G_1, G_2 etc.) corresponds with that of Table 5.1.

Table 5.1 A summary of the sources, stimuli for release and sites and modes of action of the principal gastrointestinal hormones. (↑) indicates a positive stimulus or an increase in response, (↓) indicates a negative (inhibitory) stimulus or a decrease in response.

Hormone	Source	Release stimulus						Action	
		Vagus	Protein	CHO	Fat	H⁺	Mechan.	Site	Effect
Gastrin	Pyloric antrum (Gastrin 17)	↑	↑	↑				G1) Fundus	↑H⁺ secretion (oxyntic cells) ↑Pepsin secretion (peptic cells) ↑Intrinsic factor secretion?
	Upper small intestine (Gastrin 34)				↑	↓	↑	G2) Pancreas	Weak stimulation of fluid and enzyme secretion
							↓	G3) Gall bladder	Contraction of gall bladder and bile flow
Secretin	Duodenum and upper jejunum				↑?	↑		S1) Pancreas	Profuse ↑flow of HCO₃⁻-rich juice Weak stimulation of enzyme secretion
								S2) Fundus	Inhibits H⁺ secretion, possibly by competing with gastrin for oxyntic cell receptor
								S3) Liver	↑Secretion of inorganic fraction of bile (NaCl and NaHCO₃)
								S4) Small intestine	Possible stimulation of Brunner's glands

Table 5.1 (cont.)

Hormone	Source	Release stimulus						Action	
		Vagus	Protein	CHO	Fat	H$^+$	Mechan.	Site	Effect
Pancreozymin -cholecystokinin (CCK)	Duodenum and upper jejunum		↑		↑			C1) Pancreas	Stimulation of enzyme secretion. Weak stimulation of HCO$_3$ secretion
								C2) Gall bladder	Contraction of gall bladder and relaxation of sphincter of Oddi
								C3) Fundus	Weak stimulation of acid secretion
GIP	Duodenum and upper jejunum			↑	↑			GP1) Fundus	Inhibition of acid secretion (probably relatively unimportant)
								GP2)	Stimulation of insulin secretion
Enteroglucagon	Lower small intestine and colon			↑	↑			E1)	Stimulation of insulin secretion?

gastrointestinal motility are not included in the table or figure: data relating to this and a more detailed examination of the nervous and endocrine control of the alimentary tract will be found in other books in this Series.

A number of other peptides have been isolated from mucosal extracts: some of these have had their amino acid sequences resolved, some can be measured in blood by radio-immunoassay, and all have been shown to exert effects on target tissues if injected intravenously. There remains, however, a large question mark over whether they are released under physiological conditions in amounts sufficient to produce any significant effects. The following are probably the most important of these substances.

Vasoactive intestinal peptide (VIP)

A peptide said to stimulate juice flow in the small intestine. It also depresses gastric-acid secretion.

Motilin

A peptide which causes increased gastric and intestinal contractility and may be an important factor in the control of gastric emptying.

Note

Vasoactive intestinal peptide and motilin, and other peptides not mentioned here, although not yet generally accepted as true hormones, undoubtedly are present in the mucosa and possibly the plasma of normal subjects and, in many cases, the specific cell producing a particular peptide has been defined. Moreover, in recent years, some types of clinical disorders of gastrointestinal function have been shown to be associated with overactivity of these cells and abnormally high plasma concentrations of certain of the peptides. For example, tumours which secrete VIP (vipomas) may occur in the pancreas or other sites and may cause the pancreatic cholera syndrome characterized by a profuse, watery diarrhoea.

Further reading

Bayliss, W. M. and Starling, E. H. (1902). The mechanism of pancreatic secretion. *Journal of Physiology* **28**, 325.
Bloom, S. R. (Ed.) (1978). *Gut Hormones*. Churchill Livingstone, Edinburgh.
Daggett, Peter (1981). *Clinical Endocrinology*. Edward Arnold, London.
Hobsley, M. (1981) *Disorders of the Digestive System*. Edward Arnold, London.
Sanford, P. (1981) *Digestive System Physiology*. Edward Arnold, London.

6

Neurohypophysis

Two hormones, the antidiuretic hormone (arginine vasopressin, AVP) and oxytocin, are synthesized in two specific hypothalamic nuclei and pass to the posterior pituitary gland down nerve axons—a process termed neurosecretion. The hormones are stored in the posterior pituitary gland and are from there released into the blood. The functional unit of hypothalamic nuclei, nerve-tracts and posterior pituitary gland is termed the neurohypophysis.

Arginine vasopressin promotes water reabsorption in the distal part of renal nephrons. Oxytocin causes expulsion of milk from the lactating mammary gland and uterine contractions during labour (its name is derived from the Greek for 'rapid birth').

Anatomy and microstructure of gland

The posterior pituitary gland is a downgrowth of the floor of the brain, connected to it by a stalk through which run nerve fibres (the hypothalamo-hypophysial tract) which originate in the supraoptic and paraventricular nuclei of the hypothalamus (see p.75, Fig. 7.5). The posterior pituitary gland itself contains small, modified neuroglial cells, called pituicytes, which show no cytoplasmic evidence of secretory activity. Around these cells and associated connective tissue elements are rich profusions of nonmyelinated nerve fibres from the hypothalamo-hypophysial tract whose endings are adjacent to the capillaries within the gland.

Chemistry and metabolism of hormones

Arginine vasopressin and oxytocin are peptide hormones which can be considered to be octapeptides or nonapeptides on the basis of whether cysteine is considered as one or two amino acid residues: they have closely similar structures (Fig. 6.1).

Despite their similarity in structure, the two hormones have relatively specific actions; thus, experimentally, oxytocin has less than 1 per cent of the antidiuretic action of AVP, and AVP has only 10 to 20 per cent of the effectiveness of oxytocin on the mammary gland and uterine muscle. In fact,

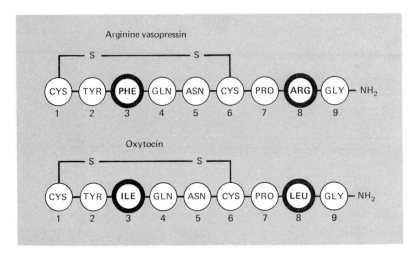

Fig. 6.1 Structures of arginine vasopressin (AVP)—antidiuretic hormone (ADH) and oxytocin.

as will be seen later, the stimuli which cause the release of each hormone are themselves sufficiently discrete not to cause significant release of the inappropriate hormone.

Neurosecretion

There is now overwhelming evidence to support the concept that the so-called posterior pituitary hormones should more accurately be designated hypothalamic hormones, since they are certainly manufactured within the neurones of two hypothalamic nuclei: AVP principally by the supraoptic nucleus (SON) and oxytocin by the paraventricular nucleus (PVN), although small quantities of oxytocin are found in the SON and likewise some AVP is found in the PVN.

The sequence of events between the synthesis of the hormones in the hypothalamic nuclei and their release into the circulation is as follows.

1. The hormones are synthesized from component amino acids within the cytoplasm of the cell bodies of the SON and PVN neurones.

Evidence
i) Small quantities of AVP and oxytocin can be demonstrated in the cell bodies of neurones in the SON and PVN respectively.
ii) Radioactive (^{38}S) cysteine injected into the CSF is incorporated within five minutes into biologically active peptides contained within secretory granules in the SON and PVN cell bodies.
iii) Isolated hypothalamus-median eminence cultures can synthesize AVP from the appropriate amino acids, while, under identical conditions, the posterior pituitary is unable to do so.

2. Secretory granules containing AVP and oxytocin, possibly bound to protein, are released from the cell bodies of the neurones of the SON and PVN

and travel down the axons to the posterior pituitary (axonal flow); the process takes about ten hours.

Evidence

i) This neurosecretory material can be readily demonstrated histologically by the Gomori technique as discrete droplets (Herring bodies) within the nerve axons.

ii) High section of the pituitary stalk causes:

a) failure of secretion of posterior pituitary hormones;
b) accumulation of neurosecretory material *above* the level of section;
c) accumulation of labelled hormone *above* the section, if ^{38}S cysteine is injected.

3. At the nerve endings within the posterior pituitary the hormones become bound to small proteins (mol.wt. about 10 000) called **neurophysins**. This binding to neurophysins is believed to aid storage within the nerve endings and also to be important in the release mechanism.

4. The hormone, together with its neurophysin, is released from the nerve ending in response to nerve impulses travelling down the axons from the SON and PVN. These axons, therefore, have a dual function. First, they act as pipes for transporting hormones from their site of synthesis in the cell body to their site of release at the nerve ending. Secondly, they transmit action potentials which trigger the release of hormone stored at the nerve endings.

Evidence Studies using the electron microscope indicate that hormones and neurophysins are released by a process of exocytosis. The mechanism is Ca^{2+}-dependent and it seems likely that the necessary Ca^{2+} enters the nerve endings as a result of depolarization caused by the arrival of the action potentials. The significance, if any, of the release of neurophysins into the circulation remains unclear. It seems certain that, at normal plasma pH, neurophysins no longer bind to AVP or oxytocin. Arginine vasopressin is probably not bound to other plasma proteins to a significant extent. It is rapidly broken down within the liver and kidney and in man has a half-life of about eight minutes.

Note The functioning of the neurohypophysis is at first sight perhaps unnecessarily cumbersome. It has, however, two great advantages. First, the posterior pituitary gland has a large capacity to *store* hormones, e.g. it contains sufficient AVP to maintain a maximum antidiuresis for about a week, whereas the SON contains less than 5 per cent of this amount. Secondly, the posterior pituitary has a rich blood supply which lies *outside* the blood–brain barrier; it therefore constitutes an ideal route for getting hormones directly and rapidly into the systemic circulation.

The two hormones will now be considered separately.

Arginine vasopressin (AVP sometimes called antidiuretic hormone)

Actions on target tissues

Kidney

In mammals, the principal target tissue for AVP is the kidney. It has long been known that crude posterior pituitary extract exerts an antidiuretic effect.

It is also now established that this is the result of an action of AVP on the distal convoluted tubules and collecting ducts of the kidney such as to make them permeable to water. Only under these conditions can osmotic movement of water occur from these parts of the nephron into the hypertonic interstitium, set up by countercurrent multiplication within the loop of Henle. There are many theories as to how AVP increases water permeability within the distal nephron, but, as a first approximation, the action of AVP appears to involve cAMP and to result in either an increase in the *number* of water-permeable 'pores' or an increase in the *size* of such 'pores'. The 'pores' remain largely hypothetical as there is no clear structural evidence for their existence.

There is also some evidence that AVP can influence intrarenal blood flow by generally increasing flow in the cortex while reducing that in the medulla. Such an action would facilitate water reabsorption by reducing flow in the vasa recta and thereby permitting more effective countercurrent multiplication within the medulla.

Blood vessels

Arginine vasopressin is a potent pressor agent. However, it appears to have no significant pressor action at physiological plasma concentrations, although during severe haemorrhage the plasma AVP concentrations are raised to within the range where pressor effects would be expected, and could therefore contribute to the other cardiovascular emergency mechanisms operating under this situation.

Effects of deficiency

Damage to the functional integrity of the neurohypophysial system which results in the severe depression or suppression of AVP secretion produces in man the chronic condition of **diabetes insipidus**, characterized by the production of large volumes (up to 10 l/day) of dilute urine (polyuria) with the secondary consequence of severe thirst and excessive fluid intake (polydipsia) (Daggett: *Clinical Endocrinology,* Chapter 6). The severity of the condition can be correlated with the extent of the damage to the neurohypophysis. If the SON is involved, or if during hypophysectomy the pituitary stalk is sectioned close to the hypothalamus such that degeneration of the supraoptic neurones takes place, the disease is severe and permanent. If, on the other hand, the stalk is sectioned close to the pituitary during hypophysectomy, there may be sufficient remaining neurosecretory function to minimize the symptoms and they are usually temporary.

It should be noted that similar symptoms to diabetes insipidus are found in the rare condition of nephrogenic diabetes insipidus, in which AVP secretion may be normal or excessive but the renal tubules are unable to respond to it. Classic diabetes insipidus can be controlled satisfactorily by administration of AVP-like substances.

Effect of excess

As would be expected, an excess of AVP causes inappropriate water retention with the consequential changes in fluid balance (Daggett: *Clinical Endocrinology*, Chapter 6).

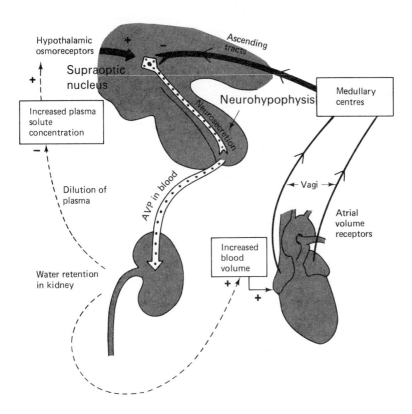

Fig. 6.2 The control of AVP secretion. (+ indicates stimulation; − indicates inhibition.)

Control of arginine vasopressin secretion (Fig. 6.2)

The rate of secretion of AVP is related to the total solute concentration or osmolality of plasma (osmoregulation) and the volume of the extracellular fluid, particularly the intravascular component (volume regulation); thus, an increase in the solute concentration or a decrease in the volume of ECF promotes AVP secretion and therefore water retention. Secretion of AVP is also increased by pain, trauma, some emotions and drugs such as nicotine and morphine. Ethyl alcohol depresses AVP secretion.

Oxytocin

Action on target tissues

Mammary gland

Oxytocin appears to play little part in the control of synthesis of milk by the lactating mammary gland, except for the still controversial possibility that it may stimulate the secretion of prolactin. Oxytocin is, however, extremely important to the mechanisms responsible for ejecting milk from the gland through the nipple. A proportion of the milk, dependent upon the species, is found in sinuses, cisterns or other dilations of the large ducts and can readily be removed passively. However, the milk within the secreting alveoli and the smaller ducts must be actively expelled. Such expulsion results from the contraction of the myoepithelial cells which are arranged around the alveoli and along the smaller ducts. The contraction appears to depend exclusively upon oxytocin and the cells are extremely sensitive to the hormone: the efferent nerves to the mammary gland play little significant part in milk ejection. Pressures of up to $10-15$ mmHg are developed in the duct system.

Uterine smooth muscle (myometrium)

As long ago as 1906, Dale demonstrated that posterior pituitary extracts caused powerful contractions of the uterus. Since then it has been established that oxytocin plays an important role in facilitating the expulsion of the fetus *once labour has begun:* it is probably not implicated in the initiation of parturition. Furthermore, there is good evidence to indicate that coitus stimulates oxytocin release and that the subsequent uterine contractions aid the transport of sperm into the Fallopian tubes.

The myometrium is composed of smooth muscle cells which can show rhythmic contractile activity due to spontaneous depolarization of the membrane potential across the cell wall (pacemaker potentials): oestrogen enhances and progesterone suppresses this activity. At the end of pregnancy, oxytocin sensitivity increases such that, once labour has begun and oxytocin secretion is stimulated by stretch of the cervix, this hormone is the principal stimulus which ensures the rapid transit of the fetus down the birth canal. At the myometrial cell level, oxytocin acts by causing a decrease in the resting membrane potential and thus an increase in the sensitivity and contractile activity of the cell, an action potentiated by oestrogens and inhibited by progesterone.

Effects of deficiency

Although oxytocin normally plays an important role in labour, present evidence suggests that it is not essential to the process. If hypophysectomy or pituitary-stalk section is performed in late pregnancy in experimental animals, parturition still occurs, although labour itself may be protracted. Moreover, in humans severe diabetes insipidus is not incompatible with normal labour in some patients, although in others labour is impaired. This variation is presumably associated with the nature of lesion causing the condition and to the extent to which the oxytocin-secretion mechanisms are involved.

The effect of hypophysectomy on the milk-ejection mechanisms cannot easily be assessed since, in the absence of prolactin, milk secretion is deficient.

Effects of excess

Oxytocin has long been used in obstetrics as a means for inducing parturition or facilitating labour. However, its effectiveness depends upon myometrial sensitivity which, in turn, is largely governed by the oestrogen/progesterone ratio. Intravenous injection of oxytocin causes a dramatic expulsion of milk from the lactating mammary gland, but this does not seem to occur when it is given during labour—presumably because lactation has not been established.

There are no clinical conditions where hypersecretion of oxytocin occurs.

Control of secretion (Fig. 6.3)

The milk-ejection reflex

Suckling, by stimulating mechanoreceptors in the nipple and within the mammary gland, promotes the release of oxytocin by a neuroendocrine reflex.

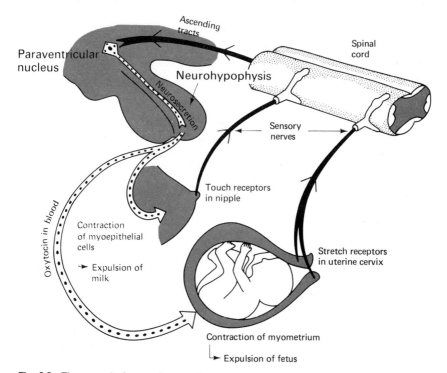

Fig. 6.3 The control of oxytocin secretion.

Afferent nerves from the mammary gland enter the spinal cord and ascending fibres connected with these synapse ultimately with these cells in the paraventricular, and, to a lesser extent, the supraoptic nuclei which initiate the neurosecretion of the hormone into the circulation. There is a latency of about one minute between suckling and the expulsion of milk.

Stimulation of the female genital tract

Mechanical stimulation of various regions of the female genital tract can elicit oxytocin release.

External genitalia

The stimulus of coitus via a neuroendocrine reflex, similar in principle to that described for the milk-ejection reflex, can cause oxytocin release, resulting in increased myometrial activity which aids sperm transport and thus increases the chance of fertilization.

Uterine cervix

Once parturition has been initiated, the fetus engages with the cervix and, by virtue of sensitive mechanoreceptors in this area, begins a neuroendocrine reflex resulting in oxytocin release. In turn, the oxytocin stimulates myometrial activity, thereby causing more oxytocin release. Positive feedback therefore results, which normally ensures that the fetus is expelled from the uterus as rapidly as possible. Consequently, the perilous time in the no-man's land between the placental attachment and a free-living existence is kept to a minimum.

Interactions between factors stimulating oxytocin release

Two points are worth remembering. First, the oxytocin release during labour helps to promote milk ejection and will, therefore aid the young at the first suckling. Secondly, and conversely, in those species producing more than one offspring, the oxytocin resulting from the suckling activity of those born early in the litter will facilitate the appearance of their siblings.

Other factors influencing oxytocin release

The normal reflex pathways from mammary gland to paraventricular neurones can be inhibited by a variety of somatic and psychological factors which constitute 'stresses'. For example, pain or physical discomfort, breast-feeding under embarrassing circumstances, fear and anger, have all been shown to depress the oxytocin released in response to suckling.

Oxytocin in the male

Oxytocin is present in the male neurohypophysis in amounts comparable with those in the female and there is some evidence that it may be released during coitus. However, oxytocin has no known function in the male animal.

Further reading

Allen, M. B. and Mahesh, V. B. (Eds.) (1978). *Pituitary: a current review.* Academic Press, New York.

Bergmann, W. and Scharrer, B. (Eds.) (1970). *Fifth International Symposium on Neurosecretion.* Springer-Verlag, New York.

Daggett, Peter (1981). *Clinical Endocrinology.* Edward Arnold, London.

Forsling, M. (1976). *Anti-diuretic Hormone,* Vol. 1. Churchill Livingstone, Edinburgh.

Forsling, M. (1978). *Anti-diuretic Hormone,* Vol. 2 Churchill Livingstone, Edinburgh.

Harris, G. W. and Donovan, B. T. (Eds.) (1966). *Pituitary Gland,* Vol. III. Pars intermedia and neurohypophysis. Butterworths, London.

7

The hypothalamus and adenohypophysis

The adenohypophysis (anterior or glandular part) of the pituitary gland is derived embryologically from buccal ectoderm. It releases six principal hormones into the systemic circulation. Five of these, adrenocorticotrophic hormone (ACTH), thyroid-stimulating hormone (TSH), the two gonadotrophic hormones—follicle-stimulating hormone (FSH) and luteinizing hormone (LH)—and finally prolactin (PRL) (also called luteotrophic hormone, LTH) have their major effects restricted to specific target organs (adrenal cortex, thyroid, reproductive organs and mammary gland respectively). The remaining hormone is growth hormone (somato-trophic hormone) which has generalized actions on many types of cell. Release of the hormones of the adenohypophysis is in part determined by feedback effects of target gland hormones, but is also subject to an over-riding modulation by specific releasing or inhibitory substances secreted by hypothalamic neurones into the portal blood vessels, which constitute the functional link between the hypothalamus and adenohypophysis. Thus, although the adenohypophysis has control over the activity of the major part of the endocrine system via the release of trophic hormones, it is itself under the influence of the hypothalamus and consequently can respond appropriately to changes in the external environment.

The influence of the hypothalamus, and thus other parts of the central nervous system, on the adenohypophysis is of such fundamental importance to any discussion of adenohypophysial activity that we shall devote the first part of this chapter to a brief consideration of the embryological, anatomical and experimental evidence which has helped clarify the details of how the hypothalamus affects the adenohypophysis.

Embryology and anatomy of the adenohypophysis

The small size of the pituitary gland belies its importance since it only weighs 600 mg in the adult human male, although it is somewhat larger in women and may grow to approach 1 g in weight at the end of pregnancy.

The parts of the pituitary gland and their anatomical relation to the hypothalamus appear complex at first sight: a situation not helped by a very confused nomenclature. The explanation for this can be supplied from an elementary understanding of the embryological development of the gland.

In the young embryo (at about six weeks in man) the roof of the mouth lies adjacent to the floor of the third ventricle of the brain and both sheets of tissue bulge toward each other (Fig. 7.1a). Eventually the upgrowth of buccal ectoderm called Rathke's pouch detaches from the roof of the mouth and begins to invaginate and grow around the funnel-shaped downgrowth of neural ectoderm, called the infundibulum (Fig. 7.1b). Finally, the tissues derived from neural ectoderm comprising the three parts of the neurohypophysis (Table 7.1) come to lie closely adjacent to the three types of tissue derived from buccal ectoderm which constitute the adenohypophysis (Table 7.1). There are wide species variations in the relative size and position of the components of the hypophysis, but the general disposition is usually as shown in Fig. 7.1c. The gland sits protected in a cup-shaped depression of the sphenoid bone at the base of the skull called the sella turcica.

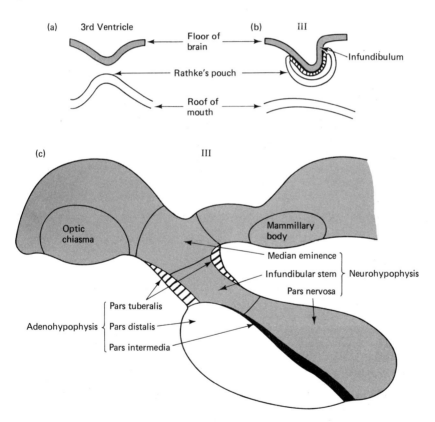

Fig. 7.1 Diagram to show the basic features of the development of the adeno- and neurohypophysis. (**a**) Early upgrowth of buccal ectoderm before Rathke's pouch has separated. (**b**) Rathke's pouch apposed to the infundibulum. (**c**) Typical mature pituitary gland (shading corresponds to that seen in (**b**).

Table 7.1   Guide to basic nomenclature of the parts of the pituitary gland and hypothalamus

Rathke's pouch (upgrowth from roof of mouth: buccal ectoderm)	Adenohypophysis	{ Pars distalis Pars tuberalis Pars intermedia	} Anterior Lobe
Downgrowth from floor of third ventricle: neural ectoderm	Neurohypophysis	{ Pars nervosa (neural lobe or infundibular process) Infundibular stem (neural stalk) Median eminence of tuber cinereum	} Posterior Lobe

Cell types in the adenohypophysis

The three regions of the mature adenohypophysis show wide differences in endocrine function and associated cellular diversity (Table 7.2). We shall not consider the pars tuberalis in view of its negligible secretary role. Moreover, the pars intermedia is indistinct in man and the functional significance of the melanotrophs remains unclear (p.78).

The pars distalis constitutes by far the largest part of the adenohypophysis and is known to secrete six hormones. It contains a variety of cell types which it is now generally accepted can be related to particular hormones on the basis of 'one cell, one hormone'.

Two principal distinctions can be made using conventional histological techniques. First, we may distinguish cells which do not readily take up dyes **chromophobes**, from those cells which do stain easily **chromophils**. Secondly, chromophils can be divided into cells which take up acidic dyes **acidophils**, and those which take up basic dyes **basophils** (Table 7.2). The designation of the secretion of particular hormones to specific cell types requires a very careful investigation of the relationship between morphological appearance and cell hormone content. The techniques used include studies of morphological changes associated with experimentally induced changes in functional activity, e.g. thyroidectomy will induce increased production of TSH, accompanied by structural changes in certain basophilic cells (thyrotrophs). The use of fluorescence-labelled antibodies to specific hormones has proved of great value in defining which cell produces which hormone, as have studies of pathological changes in pituitary function, such as dwarf mice with glands devoid of somatotrophs, or, conversely, the proliferation of these cells in conditions of excess growth hormone production (acromegaly). There remain, however, a number of points of controversy, such as whether the chromophobes are really corticotrophs or simply quiescent forms of other cells types with relatively few granules. Evidence for chromophobe ACTH hypersecreting tumours favour the former view, but, conversely, there are few chromophobe cells in the pituitary of certain species such as the pig, despite the fact that ACTH secretion is perfectly adequate in these animals: ACTH may come from basophils in such species.

Table 7.2 Cell types and their secretions in the adenohypophysis

Hormone (with abbreviation and synonyms)	Cell Type (with abbreviation and synonyms)	Staining reaction
Pars distalis		
1. Growth hormone (GH) Somatotrophic hormone (STH) Somatotrophin	Somatotroph (ST)	Acidophil
2. Prolactin (PRL) Luteotrophic hormone (LTH) Luteotrophin Mammotrophin Lactogenic hormone	Lactotroph (LT) (Mammotroph)	
3. Follicle-stimulating (FSH) hormone	Folliculotroph (FT) (FSH gonadotroph)	Basophil (particularly periodic acid-Schiff (PAS) reaction with these glycoprotein hormones)
4. Luteinizing hormone (LH) Interstitial cell-stimulating (ICSH) hormone	Luteotroph (LH gonadotroph) (Interstitiotroph) (IT)	
5. Thyroid-stimulating hormone (TSH) Thyrotrophin	Thyrotroph (TT)	
6. Adrenocorticotrophic hormone (ACTH) Corticotrophin	Corticotroph (CT)	Chromophobe? Basophil?
Pars intermedia (this is rudimentary in humans) Melanocyte-stimulating hormone (MSH) Intermedin	Melanotroph (MT)	Variable but usually weakly basophil

NB The suffix 'trophin' is preferred to the North American 'tropin' in this text.

The blood supply of the hypophysis (Fig. 7.2)

The hypophysis is supplied with arterial blood by the superior (anterior) and inferior (posterior) hypophysial arteries which are branches of the internal carotid artery. The superior hypophysial artery goes to the median eminence (1) and the infundibular stem (2) where its arterioles give rise to the primary capillary beds of the long and short portal veins respectively. The long portal veins travel to the upper and anterior parts of the pars distalis (3), while the short portal veins supply the lower, more posterior, parts (4). In some species, the inferior hypophyseal artery contributes to the primary plexus of the short portal vessels (2) and, in all species, it constitutes the major arterial supply to the pars nervosa (5).

It should be particularly noted that in almost all mammals the entire supply of arterial blood to the adenohypophysis is via the portal vessels. It is also important to realize that this blood is not simply supplying the cells with O_2 and nutrients, but is also carrying those chemicals from the hypothalamus (hypophysiotrophic hormones) which regulate adenohypophysial function (see p.71). The primary capillaries in the median eminence and infundibular stem

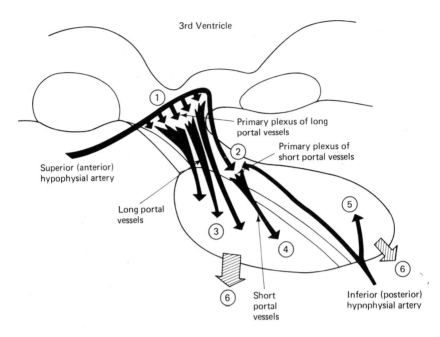

3rd Ventricle

Primary plexus of long
portal vessels

Primary plexus of
short portal vessels

Superior (anterior)
hypophysial artery

Long portal
vessels

Short
portal
vessels

Inferior (posterior)
hypophysial artery

Fig. 7.2 Diagram of the vascular organization of the pituitary (for explanation see text).

are closely invested by the endings of the neurones which synthesize and release the hypophysiotrophic hormones, while the secondary capillaries in the adenohypophysis have a discontinuous, fenestrated endothelium, presumably to facilitate passage of the hormones into the interstitial fluid. Venous blood from the pituitary passes into venous sinuses and thence to systemic veins (6).

The functional connection between the hypothalamus and adenohypophysis

All the target glands which are subject to control by anterior pituitary trophic hormones are known to change their activity in response to specific external environmental factors. Thus, thyroid secretion is stimulated by cold conditions (p.108), the adrenal cortex responds to a wide variety of 'stresses' (p.133) and gonadal activity may be altered by such factors as increasing day length, environmental temperature or coitus. Such responses are still present when the target glands are denervated or transplanted to an abnormal location and, therefore, cannot be mediated through a direct neural link to the target glands. It follows, therefore, that the change in target gland activity must reflect a change in trophic-hormone secretion from the anterior pituitary, an assumption which has been amply confirmed by measuring directly the changes in trophic-hormone secretion. External environmental changes are detected by sensory receptors which send impulses along sensory nerves to the central nervous system, from which appropriate executive commands are sent to effector tissues. How then do such commands reach the anterior pituitary? There are clearly only two possibilities; via nerves or via the circulation. The question of the nerve supply to the adenohypophysis generated great controversy in the days before the electron microscope, but this instrument has now established that what many investigators once claimed was a profuse innervation is in fact nothing more than reticulin (connective tissue) fibres. It is now accepted that, with the exception of a few autonomic fibres to blood vessels, there is no nerve supply to the adenohypophysis. Consequently, hypothalamic regulation of the adenohypophysis must be via the release of controlling factors into the circulation.

The nature of this neurovascular link was established immediately after the Second World War by the classic investigations of Harris and his co-workers, which first demonstrated the significance of the portal vessels running between the median eminence of the tuber cinereum and the anterior lobe of the pituitary (Fig. 7.2). Such vessels would be ideally suited to provide channels down which specific hypothalamic chemicals could travel and influence the anterior pituitary, but before this idea could be accepted two basic essentials had to be established. First, that flow in the vessels was from hypothalamus to pituitary and, secondly, that the integrity of the vessels was necesary for normal neural control of the anterior pituitary. After overcoming formidable technical problems, the direction of flow in mammals was demonstrated by Green and Harris, in 1949, from direct observations of the pituitary stalk in living rats. As anticipated, flow was from hypothalamus to pituitary, despite brief misgivings by Harris who, when first viewing the preparation, is said to

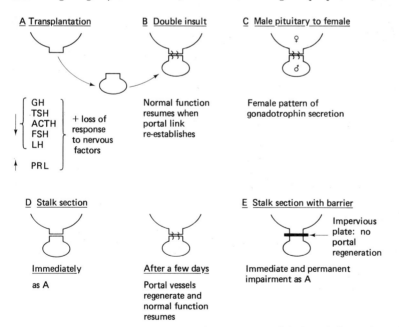

Fig. 7.3 Experiments which demonstrate the importance of the hypothalamo – hypophyseal portal vessels (for explanation see text).

have forgotten that the image in a microscope is inverted! The flow was in the right direction, but were the portal vessels the link? This was investigated by two techniques: transplanting the pituitary and sectioning the pituitary stalk. When these techniques were first developed in the early 1950s it was not possible to assay accurately the various pituitary hormones, but in the following account we will conflate the original experiments with more recent measurements of hormone changes under similar experimental conditions (Fig. 7.3).

Transplantation of the pituitary

If the pituitary is transplanted to a remote site, such as the pulp of the spleen or the anterior chamber of the eye, the graft, if successful, establishes a new blood supply and there are minimal signs of necrosis. However, two changes in adenohypophyseal function are apparent (Fig. 7.3a). First, basal secretion of all hormones except prolactin is depressed, while prolactin secretion is augmented, consequently regression occurs in the target glands. Secondly, the transplanted pituitary no longer responds to changes in central nervous activity e.g. cold no longer increases TSH secretion.

The following can be concluded from these experiments.

1. The hypothalamus influences the anterior pituitary via chemicals released into the portal vessels, the amounts released being so small as to have virtually no effect when diluted in the general circulation.

2. Hypothalamic chemicals stimulate the release of TSH, ACTH, growth hormone, FSH and LH, but inhibit the release of prolactin. (Transplantation augments prolactin secretion while depressing that of the other hormones.)

3. Hypothalamic control of the anterior pituitary is via quantitative changes in the release of specific hypothalamic chemicals into the portal vessels.

These experiments could be criticized on the grounds that the malfunction of the pituitary was simply a nonspecific consequence of the damage resulting from the transplantation. However, this objection can be elegantly refuted by removing the grafted pituitary from its remote transplantation site and replacing it back under the median eminence and thus allowing it to re-establish the direct vascular link with the hypothalamus (Fig. 7.3b). This procedure is called 'doubly insulting' the gland and it has been found that, in those second grafts which survive the procedure, normal anterior pituitary function is completely restored, thereby demonstrating that the abnormal function noted after the first graft was not due to nonspecific tissue damage. The importance of the hypothalamus in regulating anterior pituitary function is further emphasized by the observation that grafting a male pituitary under a female hypothalamus results in the female pattern of cyclical gonadotrophin secretion (Fig. 7.3c). Conversely, a female pituitary under a male hypothalamus exhibits the continuous gonadotrophin secretion characteristic of the male.

Stalk section

Another way to demonstrate the importance of the portal vessels is to section the pituitary stalk while leaving the gland *in situ* (Fig. 7.3d). Such a procedure results, as would be expected, in a rapid change in anterior pituitary function precisely comparable with that following remote transplantation (cf. Fig. 7.3a). However, within a matter of days normal function resumes spontaneously. This restoration of function provides further evidence of the importance of the portal vessels because it is found that it can be correlated with the re-establishment of the portal link by regenerating vessels. In fact, in order to establish a permanent and effective stalk section, it is necessary to interpose an impermeable plate of mica or Teflon to prevent such revascularization (Fig. 7.3e).

Hypothalamic secretions which influence the adenohypophysis

During the twenty or so years since the experimental verification of the role of the hypothalamo – hypophyseal portal vessels, a great deal of research has been devoted to the study of what precisely the hypothalamus releases into the portal vessels to influence the secretions of the anterior pituitary. In many respects these studies are amongst the most exciting in modern endocrinology; the results so far have been rewarding and many new fields of investigation have been opened up, some of which have far-reaching clinical potential. The logical first step in such work was to examine extracts of the hypothalamus and these have yielded a number of peptides which have relatively specific effects on anterior pituitary activity. These peptides were originally termed releasing or inhibitory **factors** but they have now, by convention, been given the additional status of **hormones** if their chemical structure has been characterized.

Criteria for acceptance as a hypophysiotrophic factor
Crude extracts of the hypothalamus contain a large number of biologically active substances, so rigid criteria must be imposed before any substance is accepted as a releasing or inhibitory factor. Three basic conditions should be fulfilled: first, the substance must be present in the hypothalamus and, in particular, the median eminence; secondly, it must affect the secretion of the pituitary target hormone by a *direct* effect on the gland; and, finally, there should be evidence for changes in the release of the substance commensurate with the changes in pituitary-hormone secretion. This last criterion is difficult to demonstrate in view of the problems of measuring the concentrations of hypophysiotrophic factors in peripheral blood, but this can sometimes be circumvented by measuring the concentration in portal blood (see p.75) or the changes in the hypothalamic content of the substance.

Table 7.3 summarizes the actions of the principal eight substances currently proposed, and also demonstrates the bewildering alternative nomenclature which surrounds these peptides.

Some brief remarks will now be made about particular releasing and inhibitory substances.

Thyrotrophin-releasing hormone (TRH) Thyrotrophin-releasing hormone was the first hypophysiotrophic hormone to be obtained in pure form and characterized from crude hypothalamic extracts by Schally, and a few weeks later by Guillemin. This involved research enterprise on a truly heroic scale. Thus Guillemin and his group in the USA used more than 500 tons of sheep

Table 7.3 The hypophysiotrophic substances: a table to illustrate the actions of the three hormones and five factors known to effect the pars distalis. Alternative nomenclature and abbreviations are also shown. + = Stimulation; − = inhibition.

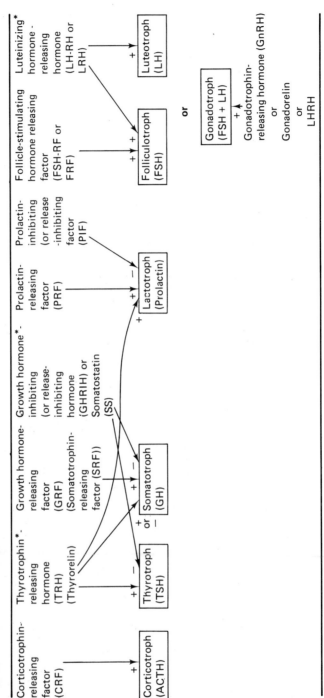

* Isolated, characterized and synthesized.

brain collected over three to four years from some 5 million sheep. Hypothalamic fragments from these brains weighed over 50 tons, but extraction of this material led to the purification of only milligram quantities of hormone, (in their definitive study in 1968, 300 000 hypothalami yielded 1.0 mg of pure TRH). Nevertheless, the effort proved worthwhile for at least three reasons.

1. Thyrotrophin-releasing hormone has been characterized chemically and has been shown to be a simple tripeptide (Fig. 7.4).

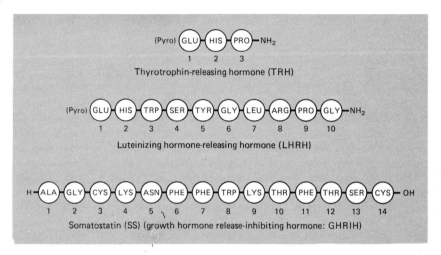

Fig. 7.4 Structure of the three hypophysiotrophic hormones so far characterized.

2. Knowing the structure, it was relatively simple to produce synthetic TRH which is proving of great value for experimental purposes and also has certain clinical applications (p.102).

3. Possession of pure TRH has allowed the development of radio-immunoassay methods for its measurement in blood and tissues.

Thyrotrophin-releasing hormone is extraordinarily potent in promoting TSH release *in vitro*, for amounts of the order of 10^{-10} mol/l are effective on the pituitary in culture, while, *in vivo*, 50 ng/kg body weight will stimulate TSH production. In addition to its stimulation of TSH secretion, TRH promotes the secretion of prolactin in all species and may either stimulate or inhibit the release of growth hormone, depending upon the species and circumstances, e.g. in man, TRH has no effect on growth-hormone secretion in normal subjects but stimulates its production in acromegaly (p.85).

Perhaps the most intriguing discovery about TRH is the fact that it is found to be widely distributed throughout the brain and spinal cord and also in the gastrointestinal tract and pancreas. This extrahypothalamic TRH has no known function, but its existence may indicate a potentially fruitful new field of study.

Corticotrophin-releasing factor (CRF) Despite the fact that, historically, the search for CRF was the first to begin, it has perhaps been the least successful.

To an extent this is a consequence of the technical problem of measuring ACTH and thereby assessing CRF activity, but further difficulties are associated with the fact that vasopressin has a potent stimulatory effect on ACTH secretion. Indeed, many workers believed that vasopressin was the physiological CRF, although this idea is now discredited by the finding of essentially normal ACTH control in a genetic strain of rats which do not synthesize vasopressin. Nevertheless, vasopressin, or a closely similar molecule, seems to be implicated in ACTH control, most probably in conjunction with at least one other peptide CRF. The situation remains confused!

Luteinizing hormone-releasing hormone (LHRH)   The LHRH has been isolated and its structure determined (Fig. 7.4). This book does not consider reproductive endocrinology in detail, so we will mention only briefly the controversy that exists about a possible FSH-releasing role of LHRH. Some authorities claim that a single anterior pituitary cell type (the gonadotroph) secretes both LH and FSH and is controlled by a single hypophysiotrophic hormone called LHRH *or* gonadotrophin-releasing hormone (GnRH) which promotes both LH and FSH release. Other workers claim that separate cells secrete FSH (folliculotrophs) and LH (luteotrophs) and that each has its own releasing hormone (FRH and LHRH respectively). Suffice it to say that the evidence is complex and that there are undoubtedly species variations.

Prolactin control   As mentioned previously (p.70), evidence from pituitary transplantation or stalk section indicates that prolactin secretion is normally tonically inhibited by hypothalamic activity and has led to a search for a prolactin-inhibitory factor (PIF). To date, no single peptide has been isolated and indeed much evidence points to the possibility that PIF may not be a peptide at all. Dopamine, a putative transmitter for the control of the release of other hypophysiotrophic hormones (p.77), has a potent prolactin-inhibitory action and is almost certain to be the PIF itself. A similar uncertainty surrounds the existence and identity of a prolactin-releasing factor (PRF). The sudden increases in prolactin release often encountered may be due either to the inhibition of PIF release and/or to the release of a specific PRF. If a PRF exists, is it identical with TRH, which has a potent stimulatory effect on prolactin secretion, or is there a separate peptide? These questions await a satisfactory answer.

Growth hormone control   Investigation of the hypothalamic factors which influence pituitary growth hormone secretion has revealed perhaps the most intriguing of all the active hypothalamic peptides—growth hormone release-inhibiting hormone (GHRIH), more usually known as somatostatin (SS). This peptide has been characterized (Fig. 7.4) and synthetic hormone is readily available. Somatostatin has been shown to inhibit GH production from pituitaries in culture and also seems to play a part in the control of GH *in vivo*; thus, basal GH secretion is abnormally high in rats treated with antibodies to SS. However, the enormous current interest in SS does not relate solely to its effect on GH, but rather to the many other effects of this peptide. These include (a) inhibition of TSH synthesis and release; (b) inhibition of basal secretion of insulin and glucagon and of the variation in the secretion of these hormones in response to many physiological stimuli (amino acids, glucose, adrenaline etc); (c) a variety of effects on the gastrointestinal tract, including inhibition of the secretion of gastric acid, secretin, pepsin, GIP, VIP and motilin; and (d) SS has also been shown to have many effects on the activity of cells in the brain, discussion of which falls beyond the scope of this book. As one might predict from its many extrapituitary effects, SS is found in, and presumably synthethized by, many tissues other than the hypothalamus, including most parts of the brain, the gastrointestinal tract and the pancreas. Somatostatin could prove to have wide clinical application and its analogues are currently undergoing evaluation for the treatment of acromegaly and a variety of gastrointestinal disorders.

Work on SS has largely overshadowed studies on growth hormone-releasing factor (GRF). That it exists is now generally accepted from studies of GH secretion from transplanted pituitaries and in animals where SS antibodies have been given, but the peptide has not been finally isolated and purified.

Mechanism of action of hypophysiotrophic substances
Much current work is directed towards an analysis of the action of hypothalamic factors/hormones on pituitary cells. The first step is interaction between the hormone and receptors in the plasma membrane of the cell. Subsequent intracellular changes appear to be largely comparable to those documented for other neural and endocrine cells in that the stimulus to secretion requires energy, causes changes in plasma-membrane permeability, is Ca^{2+}-dependent and involves cAMP. The initial effect results in the exocytotic release of previously synthesized pituitary hormones and cannot be blocked by inhibitors of protein synthesis, but recent evidence suggests that such substances will block a second, slower effect involving the synthesis of new hormone. Little is known of the details of the intracellular actions of inhibitory hormones, although there is preliminary evidence that SS may block the synthesis and expression of cAMP.

Hypophysiotrophic substances in portal blood
One of the more sophisticated approaches to the study of adenohypophysial control has been the collection and analysis of portal blood from anaesthetized rats, developed by Porter. If the pituitary gland is removed, it is possible to place a fine glass cannula against the cut stalk and to collect the blood escaping under gentle suction. A recent amazing improvement of this method has been the cannulation of single portal vessels via fine glass capillaries, a technique which can be used either to collect portal blood or to infuse substances *directly* into the blood supply to the pituitary.

Neural release of hypophysiotrophic substances We have seen that the hypothalamus, and particularly the median eminence, contains substances which can promote and inhibit the release of adenohypophyseal hormones and that these reach the gland via the portal veins. The neurones which form the tuberohypophysial tract terminate close to the primary capillaries of the portal veins and are believed to secrete the hypophysiotrophic factors/hormones. Since the hormones so far characterized are all peptides, these neurones are termed **peptidergic** (they share this nomenclature with neighbouring

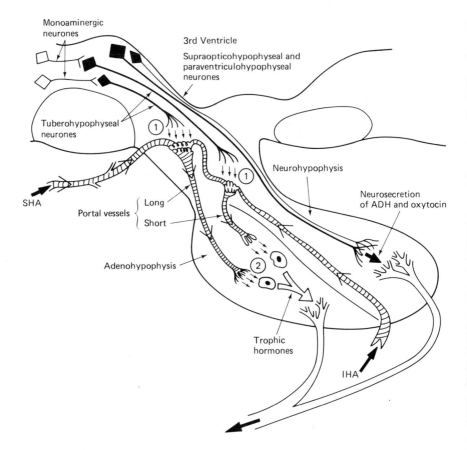

Fig. 7.5 Summary of the functional inter-relationships between hypothalamus and hypophysis. Hypophysiotrophic hormones enter the primary portal capillaries at ① and leave these vessels to influence the adenohypophyseal cells at ②. IHA = inferior hypophyseal artery. SHA = superior hypophyseal artery.

neurones secreting the neurohypophyseal peptides AVP and oxytocin). Figure 7.5 illustrates the general relations of the neurones concerned in pituitary control.

Much effort has gone into attempts to localize the cell bodies of the neurones releasing hypophysiotrophic hormones at the median eminence. In the 1960s, the main technique used was the bioassay of fragments of hypothalamus for releasing or inhibitory hormone content on the expectation that a high local content of, say, LHRH, would indicate a group of neurones synthesizing this hormone. This method met with limited success, but when used in conjunction with the results of focal damage to the hypothalamus gave some information about cellular localization. Recently, the availability of radio-immunoassay and immunocytochemical techniques has reawakened interest in this topic, —although it is too early to make definite assessments of the disposition of the cells.

The role of monoaminergic neurones   Regulation of the activity of the peptidergic neurones appears to be mediated via neurones which release either dopamine, noradrenaline or serotonin. The activity of such monoaminergic neurones is largely governed by the limbic system—the primitive part of the forebrain sometimes called the 'visceral brain'. Details of this control remain obscure, but are the subject of much research using those techniques of neuropharmacology which allow experimental manipulation of monoaminergic transmission. It is a subject in which considerable important advances can be anticipated in the near future.

Structure of adenohypophysial hormones

Studies of the structure of the six hormones of the pars distalis, the lipo-trophins and melanocyte-stimulating hormone (MSH) from the pars inter-media, have shown affinities between certain of these hormones and also with other peptide hormones of placental origin: they appear to divide into three groups (Table 7.4).

Table 7.4   Chemical affinities of adenohypophysial and placental peptides (see text).

1. **ACTH-related peptides**
    β-Lipotrophin (1–91)
    γ-Lipotrophin (1–58)
    β-MSH (37–58)
    ACTH (44–83)
    Met-enkephalin (61–65)
    α-Endorphin (61–76)
    β-Endorphin (61–91)
	Single peptide chain with certain common amino acid sequences in brackets. Peptides labelled in relation to the β-lipotrophin chain, N-terminal end is lower number.

2. **Glycoprotein hormones**
    TSH
    LH
    FSH
    HCG (human chorionic gonadotrophin)
	Two peptide chains; α chains show close similarities; β chains show marked differences. All contain carbohydrate components

3. **Somatomammotrophins**
    Prolactin
    Growth hormone
    Human chorionic somatomammotrophin
    (HCS)
	Single peptide chain with 2 or 3 internal disulphide bridges

The phylogenetic and evolutionary significance of the chemical affinities within these groups of adenohypophyseal and placental peptides remains to be resolved. However, there are often functional consequences of structural similarities. For example, pathological hypersecretion of ACTH sometimes produces abnormal pigmentation which may be attributable to the MSH-like activity of ACTH (p.129), and human chorionic somatomammotrophin (HCS), which is structurally similar to growth hormone, performs many of the actions of growth hormone during the latter half of pregnancy.

1. ACTH-related peptides

A number of closely related peptides possess a single linear peptide chain with amino acid sequences in common (Table 7.4(1)). This has led to the view that they may all be related and derive from a common precursor compound. The precursor called 'big ACTH' or 'pro-opiocortin', appears to have between 120 and 130 amino acids and, depending how it is subdivided, would produce the seven peptides listed in Table 7.4(1).

ACTH (corticotrophin)
Corticotrophin has 39 amino acids: numbers 1 to 13 are the minimum necessary to produce the biological effects of the whole molecule. Addition of numbers 14 to 20 increases the activity to that of the whole molecule. The first 24 amino acids are common to man and all other species studied: a synthetic preparation (tetracosactrin) with this structure has been found clinically to have potent biological action with minimal antigenic activity. The species-specific antigenicity resides in amino acids 25 to 33.

The actions and control of ACTH will be discussed in Chapter 9.

Melanophore (melanocyte)-stimulating hormone
The skin of certain submammalian vertebrates contains cells called melanophores which contain granules of the pigment melanin, the disposition of which influences skin coloration. The adult human pituitary contains a peptide (β-MSH) which will cause the dispersion of melanophore granules in lower vertebrates. In some mammals this peptide is secreted from the pars intermedia (hence its alternative name 'intermedin'), but in man, where this area of the pituitary is not well defined, the melanotrophs (basophils) may be found scattered in the pars distalis and also in the pars nervosa. The β-MSH has been purified from the adult human pituitary and subsequent radio-immunoassay has demonstrated it in the blood. Adrenocorticotrophic hormone has a small MSH-like activity, β-MSH has no significant ACTH activity.

The only established action of β-MSH in man is to increase melanin synthesis in the skin, which may account in part for the characteristic pallor seen in hypopituitarism. In disease states where glucocorticoid feedback inhibition of β-MSH secretion is reduced (Addison's disease), the elevated plasma MSH, together with the increased ACTH, is responsible for the hyperpigmentation seen. Secretion of β-MSH is controlled by an inhibitory factor (MIF) from the hypothalamus. Glucocorticoid feedback on the hypothalamus stimulates MIF and inhibits CRF, thus decreasing the secretion of β-MSH and ACTH respectively. In addition, β-MSH secretion may be inhibited directly by nerves from the hypothalamus.

Lipotrophins
Two fat-mobilizing peptides called β- and γ-lipotrophin have been isolated from sheep pituitaries. However, although there is no evidence yet that these peptides are secreted, their discovery may have provided essential pieces in the jigsaw puzzle of the inter-relations of single-chain peptide hormones of the adenohypophysis.

Endorphins and enkephalins

Endorphins (**end**ogenous **morphine**) are peptides which bind to opiate receptors in the brain and thus have analgesic actions. β-endorphin contains the amino acid residues of α-endorphin (61–76) plus an additional 15 at the C-terminal end (61–91): both contain the pentapeptide sequence of Met-enkephalin (61–65). This small peptide also has analgesic activity but may, in addition, be a neurotransmitter in the brain.

2. Glycoprotein hormones

The TSH, FSH, LH and HCG are each made up of two subchains (α and β) and contain carbohydrate moieties. The α chains, which have no biological activity alone, are identical or very closely similar for each hormone, whereas the β chain conveys the hormonal specificity. The β chains alone have little biological activity, but develop full potency if combined with any of the three α chains. Thus TSHα + LHβ has a luteinizing action. Although it is obviously necessary, the precise action of the α chain remains to be clarified. It has been suggested that the pituitary produces an excess of α chains and that only the synthesis of β chains is under close control.

Thyrotrophin (thyroid-stimulating hormone, TSH)

Thyrotrophin has a mol. wt. of about 20 000 and comprises an α chain of 96 amino acid residues (which, within a given species, is certainly identical with that of LH and probably also that of FSH and HCG) and a β chain of 113 amino acids: it contains about 18 per cent carbohydrate but relatively little sialic acid. The actions and control of TSH will be discussed in Chapter 8.

Follicle-stimulating hormone (FSH)

Follicle-stimulating hormone has a mol. wt. of approximately 30 000 and, once again, the β chain contains the hormonal specificity: the molecule contains a relatively large amount of sialic acid in its carbohydrate components. A detailed account of the actions of·this and other reproductive hormones will be found in other books in this series.

Luteinizing hormone (LH); intestinal cell-stimulating hormone (ICSH)

Luteinizing hormone (ICSH in the male) differs from FSH chemically in that it contains very little sialic acid: the mol. wt. is between 26 000 and 34 000 depending upon the species.

Human chorionic gonadotrophin (HCG)

This hormone is produced by the human trophoblast soon after conception. The β chain has some similarities to that of LH and there is a high sialic-acid content. Its actions resemble those of LH, although it does have some FSH-like activity.

3. Somatomammotrophins

Prolactin, growth hormone and human chorionic somatomammotrophin (HCS) (sometimes called human placental lactogen, HPL) are linear polypeptides containing internal disulphide bonds. The structure of human growth hormone has been determined as has that of HCS and, most recently human prolactin. All these peptides have close structural affinities, suggesting a common progenitor hormone.

A discussion of the function of prolactin and HCS falls beyond the scope of this book so they will not be considered further. However, the remaining hormone in this group—growth hormone—will now be considered in detail.

Growth hormone (somatotrophin)

Growth hormone (GH) is secreted by the somatotrophs of the pars distalis. It exhibits a wide range of metabolic actions which may involve virtually every type of cell. Its effects include stimulation of amino acid uptake and protein synthesis, hepatic glycogenolysis, and lipolysis within adipose tissue. Skeletal growth is promoted indirectly as a consequence of effects on bone and cartilage formation resulting from the release by GH of growth promoting peptides (somatomedins) from the liver, kidney and other tissues. Growth-hormone release is controlled by a releasing factor (GHRF) and an inhibitory hormone (GHRIH or somatostatin) secreted by the hypothalamus. Growth-hormone secretion rate reflects both metabolic requirements (increased by decreasing blood glucose or increasing blood amino acids) and neural factors (e.g. stress, circadian rhythms).

Chemistry and metabolism of growth hormone

Human growth hormone contains 191 amino acids and has a mol. wt. of about 21 500: it is a linear peptide with two disulphide bridges. Although nonprimates appear not to be species dependent in their responses to 'foreign' GH, in man only GH derived from primates is effective. Most GH used therapeutically is human autopsy material, but synthetic hormone is becoming available and some advances have been made in the use of selected fragments of nonprimate GH with high biological activity and low antigenicity.

The turnover of GH in plasma is relatively rapid: the hormone is broken down in the liver and kidney and the plasma half-life is about thirty minutes.

Action of growth hormone on target tissues

In many respects, analysis of the actions of GH presents more difficulties than that of any other hormone.

The principal reasons for this are listed below.

1. The problem of producing a specific GH deficiency. Since the adenohypophysis secretes a variety of hormones, **hypophysectomy** produces a number of sequelae which may result from the loss of hormones other than GH. In addition, many of the actions of GH itself are dependent upon or modified by the presence of other pituitary hormones. Moreover, there is no

chemical means of selectively blocking GH secretion; even somatostatin (GHRIH) affects many other hormones.

2. Many of the actions of GH are delayed and prolonged and are also difficult to study *in vitro*.

3. A wide variety of factors influence GH secretion. Such variables as nutritional status, diurnal time of sampling, species and individual differences, differences related to age, sex and emotional condition combine to make both experimental design and comparison with previous data exceedingly difficult and frustrating.

Despite the difficulties associated with the investigation of GH, much has now been established about the role of this hormone in cellular metabolism and growth. We shall examine briefly the effects of GH on protein, fat and carbohydrate metabolism, topics which will be elaborated upon in Chapter 11 when these isolated actions will be put into the general context of the endocrine control of metabolism. Finally, we shall discuss the part played by GH in the process of growth itself.

Protein metabolism

Growth hormone stimulates protein synthesis and tissue growth but the primary action of the hormone remains to be defined.

Amino acid uptake

Growth hormone stimulates amino acid uptake by cells. This effect is not secondary to increased protein synthesis since GH also stimulates the uptake of amino acids, even when protein synthesis is blocked by puromycin. Furthermore, this effect on amino acid transport is sodium dependent, whereas the GH stimulation of amino acid incorporation into protein is not.

Protein synthesis

Growth hormone stimulates the incorporation of amino acids into protein. The effect is distinct from the stimulation of cellular uptake of amino acids, although in conditions of amino acid deficiency uptake would clearly become rate limiting to protein synthesis. It remains to be established precisely how GH stimulates protein synthesis, despite many attempts to define this action in terms of nucleic acid metabolism. It seems most likely that GH increases the rate of one or several of the following steps: (a) ribosomal RNA synthesis; (b) the aggregation of ribosomes to form polysomes; (c) the attachment of RNA to ribosomes; and (d) the translation process itself.

The overall effects of GH on protein metabolism may be summarized as follows.

1. Increased protein synthesis.
2. Decreased blood amino acid concentrations.
3. Decreased urinary urea-nitrogen.
4. A positive nitrogen balance.

Fat metabolism

Growth hormone promotes the breakdown of stored fat in adipose tissue and the release of free fatty acids into the circulation. This lipolytic or adipokinetic action is completely suppressed by the administration of glucose or by feeding and is correspondingly enhanced during fasting or by hypoglycaemia. Such fat mobilization is important in providing noncarbohydrate metabolic substrate for tissues such as muscle and results in a lowering of the respiratory quotient as the fatty acids are oxidized. (The significance of the 'glucose–fatty acid cycle' will be discussed in Chapter 11.)

Details of the lipolytic action of GH remain unclear but it seems probable that it involves activation of a cAMP-sensitive lipase.

Carbohydrate metabolism

Growth hormone is diabetogenic in man, thus administration of this hormone makes clinical diabetes worse and many patients with GH-secreting tumours exhibit diabetes (see p.85). Moreover, Houssay showed, in 1924, that hypophysectomy could alleviate diabetes induced by pancreatectomy (this results from the removal of both GH and ACTH).

Growth hormone increases blood glucose concentration both by decreasing cellular uptake and utilization *and* by increasing hepatic glucose output.

> Like many of the actions of GH, its effect on the cellular uptake of glucose is complex and qualitatively different at different times. Following injection of GH there is an initial brief *increase* in glucose uptake; this is similar to the effect of insulin and serves to provide glucose needed for the re-esterification of some of the free fatty acids released by the concurrent lipolytic action of GH. This increase in glucose uptake is associated with a transient hypoglycaemia.

> The second and more obvious stage of GH action is the blockade of cellular utilization of glucose in muscle and adipose tissue by inhibition of phosphorylation. This action soon reduces entry of glucose (anti-insulin effect) and, together with the increase in hepatic glucose output, accounts for the characteristic hyperglycaemia observed during the second stage of GH action. The inhibition of glucose utilization in muscle and adipose tissue tends to conserve glucose ('glucostatic' effect) and is elegantly complementary to the increase in lipid oxidation in these tissues, made possible by the lipid-mobilizing action of GH.

Growth hormone and growth

Growth may be conveniently described as the process whereby the size of the body increases as a result of the organized addition of new tissue.

Growth hormone obtained its name as a result of the dramatic distortions of the normal postnatal growth pattern which results when it is secreted in abnormal amounts; GH deficiency being associated with dwarfism, while excessive secretion produces gigantism and acromegaly (p.85). Two general points must be remembered about the effects of GH on growth. First, the effects cannot be attributed entirely to a combination of the diverse metabolic effects of the hormone described above, although these effects will clearly play a role in the control of growth. Secondly, GH itself is not responsible for all aspects of growth. It is certainly necessary for overall body growth after the immediately postnatal period (fetal and early neonatal growth are relatively independent of GH), but many other aspects of growth, including regenerative growth and wound healing, hair growth and certain of the pubertal changes in the configuration of the body, do not require GH.

Bone growth is secondary to the formation of cartilage; this is well shown in the long bones where growth occurs initially by the deposition of cartilage at the epiphyseal plates at the ends of the bone: a convenient experimental index of this process, and thus of the rate of bone formation, can be obtained by measuring the rate of incorporation of radioactive sulphate into chondroitin sulphate in such cartilage segments *in vitro*. Daughaday and co-workers, in the late 1950s, who used this preparation in an attempt to analyse the mode of action of GH, provided the first evidence for an indirect control of bone growth, when they failed with GH to stimulate sulphate incorporation in cultures of cartilage from hypophysectomized rats. However, they found that the plasma of either normal animals or hypophysectomized animals treated with GH for a few hours *did* stimulate sulphate incorporation, even though GH itself did not. They surmized therefore, that GH promoted the formation of a second humoral factor which acted on the cartilage: this substance they called initially 'sulfation factor'.

Progress since this basic research may be summarized as follows.

1. The original 'sulfation factor' has been shown to have a variety of effects other than simple sulphation. These include stimulation of thymidine incorporation into DNA and thus cell replication, incorporation of leucine into RNA and the conversion of proline into collagen hydroxyproline.

2. These, and other actions originally attributed to the single 'sulfation factor', are now known to be mediated by a family of peptides called **somatomedins**.

3. Three somatomedins have been isolated so far; somatomedin A is a neutral peptide (mol. wt. 7000) probably identical with the 'sulfation factor'; somatomedin B is an acidic peptide (mol. wt. 5000) whose effects include the promotion of thymidine incorporation into DNA; somatomedin C promotes both sulphate incorporation and thymidine uptake.

4. Notwithstanding the isolation of these three peptides, it seems that *in vivo* they are normally associated with a larger binding protein in serum; this is sometimes called 'big somatomedin' and has a mol. wt. of 50 000.

5. From the results of perfusion studies, it seems that somatomedins are produced in the liver and possibly, but to a much lesser extent, in the kidney.

6. Somatomedins share many of the properties of insulin and may sometimes even compete with insulin for common receptors. This insulin-like action is of course not suppressed when animals are treated with specific anti-insulin antibodies, and is thus sometimes called 'non-suppressible insulin-like activity' (NSILA). Since NSILA is GH dependent it may explain the mechanism of those aspects of GH actions which resemble those of insulin, such as the general anabolic effects.

Effect of growth hormone deficiency

Depressed secretion of GH is most commonly encountered in cases of pituitary insufficiency (hypopituitarism) and its effects are therefore difficult to separate from the associated failure of other pituitary hormones (Daggett: Clinical Endocrinology, Chapter 6). In such cases it is a reasonable approximation to say that few, if any, of the consequences of hypopituitarism in the *adult* can be attributed specifically to a lack of GH. However, in childhood and adolescence, deficient GH secretion can produce profound impairment of growth.

Growth hormone must play only a small part in controlling growth in early life because pituitary dwarfs grow virtually normally until they are between 2 and 4 years old. Thereafter, until puberty, GH is the prime determinant in the rate of growth of the long bones and hence the increase in stature. During this period, individuals deficient in GH grow at less than half the normal rate, although, since epiphysial closure is delayed, growth continues for longer than in normal subjects.

Rarely, dwarfism can be attributed to an isolated failure of GH secretion transmitted genetically as a recessive defect. Small stature can result from abnormalities in GH metabolism other than deficient secretion. Thus, GH levels are normal in African pygmies so their small stature must be in part a consequence of other factors, either a slightly abnormal and less effective GH molecule, or a failure of peripheral response to GH or perhaps deficient somatomedin production. This last possibility is in accord with the observation that certain dwarf children have high GH levels but low somatomedin concentrations—Laron dwarfism (cf. p.87).

Effect of growth hormone excess

Hypersecretion of GH occurs most commonly as the direct result of acidophil tumours of the anterior pituitary. If excessive secretion of GH occurs before the epiphyses have closed, gigantism will result: in adults the result is acromegaly.

Gigantism

This is a rare condition where excessive growth of an essentially normal pattern leads to extremely large individuals with normal bodily proportions (Daggett: *Clinical Endocrinology*, Chapter 6). The growing period is lengthened since there is a delay in epiphysial closure and indeed the most famous recent giant was still growing at the time of his death at the age of 22, with a height of 8ft 11ins (2.72 m): in fact almost all 'extreme' giants tend to die in early adulthood as a result of progressive debility, infection, or as a consequence of other pituitary abnormalities.

Acromegaly

If GH oversecretion occurs after the epiphyseal plates have fused, the abnormal growth manifests itself in the extremities (acromegaly = 'large extremities'). Acromegalics have large, elongated heads with prominent jaws and coarsened facial features (Daggett: *Clinical Endocrinology*, Chapter 6). The hands and feet are enlarged and spade-like, while other skeletal abnormalities tend to induce arthritis. Overgrowth of soft tissues leads to enlargement of organs such as the spleen, pancreas, thyroid and kidneys, while other symptoms may be related to pressure exerted by the enlarged pituitary itself on, for example, the optic chiasma; as mentioned previously, there is also a tendency towards diabetes.

Control of growth hormone secretion

In recent years, the development of sensitive radio-immunoassays for GH have revealed a number of unexpected findings about the rate at which it is secreted. First, the plasma concentrations show little correlation with age and stage of postnatal growth; comparable values are found in infancy and old age. Secondly, the half-life of GH is surprisingly short and can be measured in minutes, and, finally, the rate of secretion can fluctuate suddenly producing dramatic peaks in plasma concentration lasting for only a few minutes: the reason for this 'episodic' secretion remains to be explained.

A variety of factors, both chemical and neural, influence the secretion of GH, all of which depend on the integrity of the hypothalamo-pituitary connection and almost all of which involve the brain adrenergic system (Fig. 7.6). Thus, α-adrenergic pathways serve to stimulate GH release (blocked by

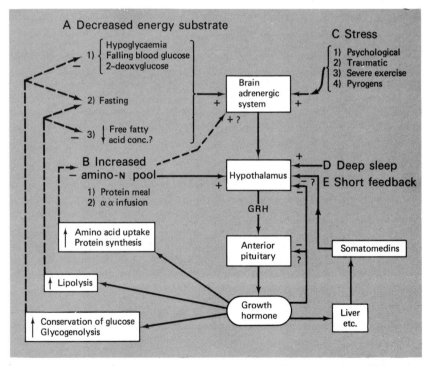

Fig. 7.6 The control of growth-hormone secretion (see text). ($\alpha\alpha$ = amino acids.)

phentolamine), while β-adrenergic pathways appear to inhibit GH release (blocked by propranolol).

The factors which influence GH secretion will now be reviewed briefly. (The lettering and numbering of the following subsections corresponds with that in Fig. 7.6.)

A. Decreased energy substrate

1. A low or falling blood glucose concentration

The secretion of GH in response to intracellular glucose deficiency is a particularly appropriate homeostatic response, since GH increases lipid mobilization and utilization, while at the same time decreasing peripheral glucose utilization and thereby protecting the brain from glucose deficiency (see Fig. 11.2).

> The stimulus appears to work by the reduction of the intracellular availability of glucose, since 2-deoxy-D-glucose, which blocks intracellular glucose metabolism, is also effective. The receptors for this effect seem, from the evidence of localized lesions and microinjections of glucose, to be in the lateral hypothalamus. They effect secretion of GHRH indirectly via the brain adrenergic system, since α-adrenergic blockade decreases and β-adrenergic blockade potentiates the GH response to hypoglycaemia.

2. Fasting

Although there have been reports of a slow rise in plasma GH during fasting, and the glucose-conserving and fat-mobilizing actions of this hormone would be peculiarly suitable under these circumstances, it seems unlikely that GH is the prime metabolic regulator during fasting. Nevertheless, the 'back-up' provided by GH is probably important in supplementing the insulin-glucose feedback which appears to be the pre-eminent factor among the many endocrine changes seen during fasting (p.153).

3. Decline in plasma free fatty acids (FFA)

One of the major effects of GH concerns the mobilization of stored fat and the consequent elevation of plasma FFA concentrations. Many workers have therefore looked for a negative feedback control of GH secretion by FFA in plasma. However, while it is established that increased FFA concentrations suppress GH secretion (e.g. that induced in response to insulin hypoglycaemia), the converse, a significant stimulation of GH by falling or low FFA concentrations, has yet to be convincingly demonstrated.

B. Increased plasma amino acids

Growth hormone produces a marked acceleration both of amino acid uptake by cells and of subsequent protein synthesis. This anabolic effect would lead one to expect the secretion of GH in response to an increase in circulating amino acids. Such a stimulation of GH secretion can be demonstrated to follow the intravenous infusion of certain amino acids, but the response to amino acids entering the circulation from digested protein is less clear-cut, in view of the concurrent changes in plasma glucose and FFA (postingestive hormonal changes will be discussed at length in Chapter 11).

In contrast to the effects of carbohydrate and fat on GH secretion, the effects of amino acids are substantially independent of the brain adrenergic system.

C. Stress

A wide variety of physical and psychological stresses promote GH secretion. Examples include anxiety concerning a dental visit, venepuncture, pain, surgery, strenuous exercise and bacterial pyrogens. In each case, pharmacological methods have shown that the brain adrenergic system is involved in the response. The role of the increased GH secretion induced by such stresses is not known.

D. Deep sleep

Marked elevations in GH secretion are associated with periods of deep sleep. The significance of the phenomenon is not understood, although it has been suggested that the brain is 'maintaining and responding to the nutritional state of the body'. What precisely this suggestion implies remains equally unclear! The response during deep sleep is independent of the brain adrenergic system.

E. Short feedback control

Unlike TSH, ACTH and the gonadotrophins, GH has no target gland and therefore there can be no feedback control by target-gland hormones. However, there is evidence that GH may influence its own secretion by exerting an inhibitory effect on the release of GHRH. For example, pretreatment with GH lowers pituitary GH content and suppresses the GH response to insulin-induced hypoglycaemia.

> Although it is generally assumed that these effects are due to the 'short feedback' effect of GH itself on the hypothalamus or pituitary, it could possibly also be due to an indirect effect of the metabolic effects of GH or even to a feedback via somatomedins. Evidence for the latter possibility comes from the observation that there are high plasma GH levels in children unable to produce somatomedins (Laron dwarfs).

Conclusion

The secretion of GH can be modulated by a variety of neural and bloodborne factors, but in only a few cases can one discern a 'tactical' purpose for the effect. Indeed, apart from the obvious lack of body growth resulting from GH deficiency, there are little, if any, significant physiological consequences associated with the absence of this hormone, with the exception of an increased sensitivity to insulin.

Effects of anterior pituitary deficiency

Generalized loss of anterior pituitary function (panhypopituitarism) may result from a variety of causes including damage due to impairment of the blood supply, therapeutic x-irradiation, bacterial infection, trauma, surgical hypophysectomy, or the presence of large nonsecretory tumours: rarely, the pituitary is congenitally absent or grossly abnormal. Recently, the availability of releasing hormones, such as TRH, has enabled the demonstration that some causes of apparent failure of the anterior pituitary were, in fact, secondary to the hypothalamic malfunction. However, the pituitary has a large reserve and therefore noticeable impairment of function only results when the major part of the gland has been eliminated; in dogs at least 70 per cent of the gland must be removed before gonadotrophic secretion is affected, 90 to 95 per cent before affecting TSH and virtually 100 per cent before ACTH secretion suffers.

Total removal of the adenohypophysis in man results in death, unless appropriate hormone replacement therapy is instituted. In practice, the limiting factor is the adrenocortical insufficiency resulting from the loss of ACTH. Provided glucocorticoids are administered, the danger of acute crises is thus largely removed, and replacement of thyroid and gonadal hormones can be instituted with less urgency. Replacement therapy using target-gland hormones is preferable to attempts to use pituitary hormones in view of the problems the latter generate in terms of antigenicity, cost and the short duration of their action.

Loss of the entire adenohypophysis results in adrenal atrophy and consequences appropriate to glucocorticoid deficiency (p.129). It should be noted that aldosterone secretion is largely unaffected so that electrolyte and water balance is less upset than in acute adrenal failure. The symptoms of thyroid deficiency which occur resemble those of myxoedema (p.101) and require similar treatment. Gonadotrophin deficiency results in gonadal atrophy, amenorrhea, and loss of libido and some of the secondary sexual features. Loss of growth hormone in young individuals impairs growth and in adults may result in protein loss. There is a tendency towards hypoglycaemia which can be attributed to deficiency of ACTH and thus glucocorticoids, and also to the lack of growth hormone: loss of growth hormone also predisposes to insulin hypersensitivity due to the loss of its anti-insulin effects. The preceding discussion concerns the general consequences of hypophysectomy, there are, however, recognized syndromes associated with the more or less specific loss of particular adeno-hypophyseal hormones: these will be considered in more detail in the *Clinical Endocrinology* text.

Effects of anterior pituitary overactivity

There are, of course, no circumstances when all the adenohypophyseal hormones are present in excess, but there are well-documented cases of tumours causing hypersecretion of individual hormones. Some of these will be discussed in the appropriate chapters: growth hormone excess (p.85); ACTH excess (p.130); TSH excess (p.102). Hypersection of FSH and LH by gonadotrophin-secreting tumours is extremely rare, while tumours secreting prolactin are common and may cause galactorrhea (persistent or abnormal lactation).

Further reading

Allen, M. B. and Mahesh, V. B. (Eds.) (1978). *Pituitary: a current review*. Academic Press, New York.

Costa, E. and Trabucchi, M. (Eds.) (1977). Endorphins. *Advances in biochemical psychopharmacology* 18. Raven Press, New York.

Daggett, Peter (1981). *Clinical Endocrinology*. Edward Arnold, London.

Elde, R. and Hökfelt, T. (1979). Localization of hypophysiotrophic peptides and other biologically active peptides within the brain. *Annual Review of Physiology* 41, 587.

Greep, R. O. and Astwood, E. B. (1974). Endocrinology: Handbook of Physiology, Vol. IV. *The Pituitary Gland and its Neuroendocrine Control*, Part I. American Physiological Society, Washington.

Greep, R. O. and Astwood, E. B. (1974). Endocrinology: Handbook of Physiology, Vol. IV. *The Pituitary Gland and its Neuroendocrine Control*, Part 2. American Physiological Society, Washington.

Harris, G. W. and Donovan, B. T. (Eds.) (1966). *Pituitary Gland, Vol. I. Anterior pituitary*. Butterworths, London.

Harris, G. W. and Donovan, B. T. (Eds.) (1966). *Pituitary Gland, Vol. II. Anterior pituitary*. Butterworths, London.

Jeffcoate, S. L. and Hutchinson, J. S. M. (1978). *The endocrine hypothalamus*. Academic Press, London.

Krulich, L. (1979). Central neurotransmitters and the secretion of prolactin, GH, LH and TSH. *Annual Review of Physiology* 41, 603.

Luft, R. and Hall, K. (Eds.) (1975). *Somatomedins and some other growth factors*. Advances in metabolic disorders, Vol. 8. Academic Press, New York.

Schally, A. V., Coy, D. H. and Meyers, C. A. (1978). Hypothalamic regulatory hormones. *Annual Review of Biochemistry* 47, 104.

Suzuki, M., Kondo, Y., Takahashi, T. and Yukitake, Y. (Eds.) (1978). *Brain monoamines and the control of endocrine secretion*. 15th Gumna Symposium, Institute of Endocrinology, Maebashi.

Watkins, W. B. (1977). *Hypothalamic releasing factors*, Vol. I. Churchill Livingstone, Edinburgh.

Watkins, W. B. (1978). *Hypothalamic releasing factors*, Vol. II. Churchill Livingstone, Edinburgh.

8

The thyroid gland

The thyroid gland secretes two iodine-containing hormones, thyroxine (T_4) and tri-iodothyronine (T_3), and the peptide calcitonin (CT). Thyroxine and T_3 stimulate oxidative metabolism in most cells and have a wide spectrum of other actions including effects on carbohydrate, fat and protein metabolism, growth processes and central nervous function. Thyroxine and, to a lesser extent, T_3 have a protracted action, partly attributable to long half-lives, and usually there is a marked latent period between administration of the hormone and its effect. Thyroid secretion is regulated by thyroid-stimulating hormone (TSH) from the adenohypophysis. The secretion of TSH is modulated by thyrotrophin-releasing hormone (TRH) from the hypothalamus in relation to factors such as environmental temperature and stress: TSH and perhaps TRH are subject to feedback inhibition by unbound thyroid hormones in the plasma. Calcitonin serves to lower Ca^{2+} concentration in blood by increasing bone calcium stores and will be discussed in a subsequent section.

Anatomy and microstructure

Phylogenetically and embryologically the vertebrate thyroid is associated with the gastrointestinal tract. Its evolutionary precursor is probably the protochordate endostyle, which secretes mucus into the gut but which can concentrate iodide and produce iodinated amino acids identical with those seen in the vertebrate thyroid. The human thyroid begins to develop about four weeks after conception as a thickening and then a diverticulum from the floor of the pharynx. It moves down the neck while developing its final bilobed shape and breaking the thyroglossal duct, its connection with the pharynx. The lobular, follicle-containing, mature form of the gland appears by the last third of gestation.

In the normal adult the gland weighs about 25 g and its two lobes, connected by an isthmus, closely invest the trachea. It has a high blood flow (about 5 ml/g per minute), only exceeded by that to the lungs and carotid body: the blood supply is illustrated in Fig. 2.1. It also has a rich autonomic innervation from the vagus and cervical sympathetic trunks, although the function of these nerves is unclear since denervation or transplantation to a remote site does little to alter thyroid activity.

The gland is divided, by ingrowth of its connective tissue capsule, in lobules within which are found clusters of follicles or acini: there are over 1 million follicles in the human thyroid. Each follicle is approximately spherical and comprises a single layer of cells surrounding a clear mucus-like fluid—the colloid (thyroglobulin). In active glands the follicles are small and the colloid is reduced since the follicular cells increase in size and erode the colloid adjacent to their apical surfaces, while in quiescent glands the follicles are enlarged and distended with colloid and the cells are flattened. Follicular cells are similar to other secretory cells in possessing a well-developed endoplasmic reticulum and Golgi apparatus but, in addition, there are numerous microvilli on the apical surface of the cell which extend into the colloid. Active cells increase in height and develop their secretory apparatus, while colloid droplets and more lysosomes become apparent and some of the microvilli elongate into pseudopodia. These changes are related to the unique ability of the follicular cell to function in three modes: first, as an **exocrine** cell by secreting products into the follicular lumen; second, as an **absorptive** cell by pinocytosing these secretions back into the cell; and finally, as a true **endocrine** cell by releasing hormones directly into the blood stream (see below).

Chemistry and metabolism of hormones

Thyroxine and tri-iodothyronine, the principal hormones secreted by the thyroid, are iodinated amino acids. The essential synthetic steps and detailed structure of the hormones and their precursors are illustrated in Fig. 8.1. It is necessary, however, to follow hormone synthesis in more detail and in particular to relate it to events within the thyroid itself. We shall undertake this by looking at each stage of the synthesis and release of T_4 and T_3 in sequence, using the same numbering as in Fig. 8.2.

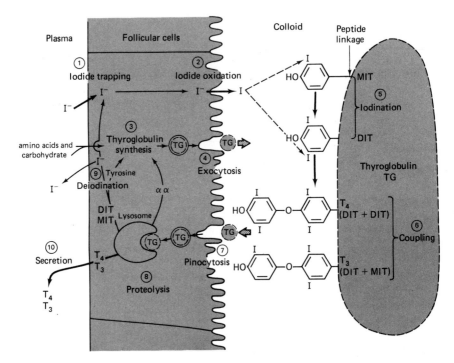

Fig. 8.2 Diagram to illustrate the synthesis and secretion of T_4 and T_3 by a follicular cell (see text).

a) Synthesis and release

1. *Iodide trapping*
Iodide from food and drinking water is absorbed by the small intestine as inorganic iodide. As long as the daily intake does not fall below about $100-150$ μg for long periods, iodine does not constitute a limiting factor for thyroid function, although chronic iodine deficiency does lead to hypothyroidism (p.101).

Iodide is concentrated by the thyroid from the blood perfusing it. The iodide 'trap' is extremely efficient in capturing iodide as the thyroid to serum-free iodide concentration ratio (T/S ratio) is normally about 25. The efficiency of the pump is largely dependent upon TSH; thus, after hypophysectomy, the T/S ratio may fall to less than 5, while with excess TSH or in iodine deficiency it can exceed 250. The long-acting thyroid stimulator (LATS) also stimulates thus mechanism (p.102).

Iodide crosses the basal membrane of the follicular cells against both a concentration gradient and an electrical gradient since the inside of the cells has a negative potential of $40-50$ mV. This active transport is known as the iodide pump and is a carrier-mediated, energy-requiring mechanism linked to the $Na^+ - K^+$-dependent ATPase system.

The trap is blocked by certain anions such as perchlorate and thiocyanate which are believed to act by *competing* with iodide for the carrier mechanism.

2. *Iodide oxidation*
Before it can enter into organic combination, iodide must be converted into free iodine ($2I^- \rightarrow I^2 + 2E$). This oxidation occurs at the microvilli under the action of a membrane-bound peroxidase enzyme with hydrogen peroxide acting as the electron acceptor. Free iodine is therefore released at the cell/colloid interface, which is presumably where the subsequent iodinations occur. The thyroid peroxidase enzyme can be inhibited by drugs such as propylthiouracil (PTU).

3. *Thyroglobulin synthesis*
Thyroglobulin is a glycoprotein (mol.wt. 660 000) and is synthesized within the follicular cells in the usual way by the assembly of polypeptide chains on the ribosomes and then the final addition of the carbohydrate moieties. At this stage the protein is sometimes called 'prethyroglobulin' as it is not yet iodinated and 'mature'.

4. *Exocytosis*
Membrane-bound vesicles containing uniodinated thyroglobulin pass from the follicular cells through the apical cell membrane into the colloid by the process of exocytosis (reverse pinocytosis).

5. *Iodination*
Free iodine, formed as in 2, rapidly becomes attached at the 3 position (see Fig. 8.1) of tyrosyl groups held by peptide linkages to the thyroglobulin molecules: this process forms monoiodotyrosine (MIT). A further iodination of MIT at the 5 position yields di-iodotyrosine (DIT).

6. *Coupling*
The organic binding of iodine to form MIT and DIT is followed by the coupling of two iodinated tyrosine molecules via an ether linkage to form the hormonally active iodothyronines; thus $DIT + DIT \rightarrow T_4$ + alanine or $MIT + DIT \rightarrow T_3$ + alanine (see Fig. 8.1). The actual reactions are much more complex than Fig. 8.1 would suggest, and probably involve a peroxidase, which may be the same as that responsible for the earlier oxidation of iodide.

7. *Pinocytosis*
Iodinated (or 'mature') thyroglobulin is the storage form of the thyroid hormones: the T_4 and T_3 residues still attached to the thyroglobulin are stored in the lumen as part of the colloid. In fact, the thyroid contains up to two weeks' supply of hormone, which is a much greater reserve than that found in any other endocrine gland. The proportions of iodinated compounds in the colloid are approximately one-quarter as MIT, one-third as DIT, one-third as T_4 and the remainder as T_3 and traces of other compounds such as reverse T_3 ($3,3',5',T_3$).

The first stage of hormone secretion is the pinocytotic ingestion of the peripheral colloid by the phagocytotic action of the microvilli and the pseudopodia which grow from the apical membrane of the follicular cells. This process is stimulated by TSH.

8. *Proteolysis*
After pinocytosis the thyroglobulin appears in the apical cytoplasm as 'colloid droplets'. These fuse with lysosomes to form phagolysosomes, within which proteolytic degradation of the thyroglobulin occurs. This process releases amino acids (which may be reincorporated into new thyroglobulin), MIT and DIT (which are subsequently deiodinated) and T_4 and T_3 (which are secreted).

9. *Deiodination*
A cytoplasmic deiodinase catalyses the removal of iodide from MIT and DIT; the iodide and tyrosine released may either leave the cells or be recycled.

10. *Secretion*
Thyroxine and T_3 are relatively immune to deiodination, although partial deiodination of some of the T_4 to form the more biologically active T_3 may take place, particularly during iodine deficiency. Secretion of T_4 and T_3 occurs by diffusion down the concentration gradient from cell to plasma. This gradient may be as high as 100:1 and is of course aided by the binding of free

Table 8.1   Factors influencing thyroid function (numbers as Fig. 8·2)

	Stimulated	Inhibited by
1. Iodide trapping	TSH LATS (TSAb) Iodide deficiency	Hypophysectomy Perchlorate Thiocyanate Quabain Iodide excess
2. Iodide oxidation	TSH?	Hypophysectomy Thiocyanate
3. Thyroglobulin synthesis	TSH	Hypophysectomy Inhibitors of protein synthesis
5. Iodination and 6. Coupling	TSH	Thiouracil, carbimazole
7. Pinocytosis	TSH	Hypophysectomy
8. Proteolysis	TSH	Hypophysectomy
9. Deiodination		Dinitrotyrosine
10. Secretion	TSH (perhaps secondary to previous effects)	Hypophysectomy

TSH = Thyroid-stimulating hormone (thyrotrophin); LATS = long-acting thyroid stimulator;
TSAb = thyroid-stimulating antibodies.

T_4 and T_3 to plasma proteins. In euthyroid (normal) subjects the ratio of T_4:T_3 secreted is 20–30:1. The MIT, DIT and thyroglobulin are not normally secreted, although thyroglobulin may enter the blood in disease states, especially thyroid carcinoma.

The ways in which processes 1–10 as described above can be stimulated or inhibited are summarized in Table 8.1.

b) Transport of thyroid hormones in blood

It is important to realize two points about the transport of T_4 and T_3 in blood.

1. Virtually all ($>$99.5 per cent) of the hormone is protein bound.
2. Only the free (unbound) hormone is biologically active.

In view of these facts, it is clear that the binding of T_4 and T_3 to plasma proteins is of extreme relevance to thyroid activity and that it will be necessary to discuss the purpose and the nature of protein binding.

Both T_4 and T_3 are essentially iodinated amino acids and, as such, in the absence of protein binding would be rapidly filtered by the kidney and lost in the urine, but by being bound to proteins of high mol.wt. the hormones are neither filtered by the glomeruli nor do they cross other capillary walls readily. Consequently they are effectively retained within the vascular system. Furthermore, the existence of a huge supply of bound hormone in the blood in equilibrium with free hormone provides an immediate 'buffer' to counteract the effects of rapid fluctuations either in the supply of or demand for free hormone. It will be seen from Table 8.2A that only a minute proportion of the total T_4 and T_3 in the plasma is in the free form.

In man, T_4 is bound to three types of plasma protein, as shown in Table 8.2B. The characteristics of protein binding have been demonstrated quantitatively by the use of radio-iodinated T_4 and T_3 in conjunction with

Table 8.2 Carriage of thyroid hormones in blood. Normal values (approximate)

A.	Total	Percentage free	Absolute concentration free
T_4	50–150 nmol/l (4–12 µg/dl)	0.03	11–23 pmol/l (1.2–3.6 ng/dl)
T_3	0.9–2.8 nmol/l (0.06–0.18 µg/dl)	0.3	3–8 pmol/l (approx.) (0.2–0.5 ng/dl approx.)

B Binding proteins

	Concentration (mg/dl)	Binding affinity	Saturation capacity (µg/100 ml)	Actual binding T_4	Actual binding T_3
TBG	2	Very high	20	75%	75%
TBPA	25	Low	200	15%	0%
Albumin	4500	Very low	—	10%	25%

paper or gel electrophoresis. From such studies it has been found that about 75 per cent of both T_4 and T_3 are bound to thyroxine (or thyronine)-binding globulin (TBG). Thyroxine-binding globulin is an α-2-globulin of approximate mol.wt. 60 000. It appears to have one thyronine-binding site per molecule and has a very high affinity for both T_4 and T_3. Thyroxine-binding prealbumin (TBPA) has a much lower affinity for T_4 than TBG, so, although it is present in higher concentration than TBG, it only accounts for 15 per cent of T_4 binding: T_3 does not bind to TBPA. Serum albumin, which is present in much higher concentration than TBG and TBPA, has an extremely low affinity for T_4 and so accounts only for 10 per cent of the binding: about 25 per cent of T_3 is also bound to albumin. Clinically, an approximate index of circulating T_4 can be obtained from measurement of the protein-bound iodine (PBI) (T_3 constitutes less than 5 per cent of the total PBI), although the availability of radio–immunoassays for T_4 means that direct measurements have now superseded the PBI technique.

Fluctuations in plasma protein binding may lead to large variations in the *total* plasma T_4 and T_3 but, since the *free* hormone concentration is the subject of feedback regulation via TSH (p.106), changes in total plasma T_4 and T_3 do not (after equilibration) represent changes in thyroid status. Examples of situations where binding is altered are the reduction after treatment with salicylates which compete with T_4 for binding sites on TBPA and the increase resulting from the increase in plasma-binding proteins during pregnancy or caused by oestrogen therapy.

c) Metabolism of thyroid hormone

The use of radioactive T_4 and T_3 has made possible quantitative studies of metabolism of these hormones: Fig. 8.3 represents in diagrammatic form the various pathways involved and should be studied in conjunction with the following summary, which is similarly numbered. (*NB* All values quoted below are approximations.)

1. The thyroid secretes a total of $80-100$ μg of T_4 and T_3/day. The ratio of T_4:T_3 is normally approximately 20:1.

2. In plasma, free hormone is in equilibrium with protein-bound hormone. (Only about 1/3000 of the T_4 is free). Free T_4 and T_3 enter cells of the liver and other tissues.

3. Of the T_4 in tissues, 80 per cent is deiodinated.

4. About half of the deiodinated T_4 joins the tissue pool of T_3: *N.B.* T_4 is the source of about 90 per cent of the T_3 available to tissues (see 6). The iodide released from deiodination of the remaining T_4 is excreted in the urine or recirculated to the thyroid.

5. About one-third of the T_4 leaving the plasma is excreted in the bile, either free or after conjugation in the liver with glucuronate or sulphate. A proportion of the free or conjugated T_4 entering the gut in the bile is reabsorbed (the **enterohepatic circulation** of T_4), the rest is lost in the faeces.

6. The daily disposal rate of T_3 is 30 μg, of which 27 μg are derived from T_4 and only 3 μg from thyroid secretion of T_3.

7. & 8. About 80 per cent of T_3 is deiodinated and 20 per cent is lost in the faeces (see 4 and 5 above).

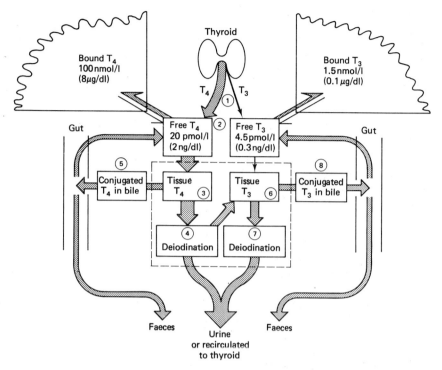

Fig. 8.3 The metabolism of T_4 and T_3: width of arrows indicates approximate relative magnitude of fluxes (see text).

In normal adults, the daily peripheral turnover of T_4 represents about 10 per cent of the extrathyroidal pool: the hormone thus has a half-life of six to seven days. The turnover of T_3 is much more rapid (60 per cent per day) and the half-life is about one day.

The actions of thyroid hormones

Information about the actions and effects of thyroid hormones has been gained primarily from studies of human and animal subjects with either overactive or depressed thyroid function (hyper-and hypothyroid conditions). Additional information has been obtained from observing the effects of the hormones on organs or tissues *in vitro* and from detailed biochemical studies of their cellular and subcellular actions. Much recent interest has been focussed on the suggestions discussed previously, that T_3 is probably the biologically active agent and that T_4 may be little more than a prohormone and a stable and regulated source of T_3. Certainly T_3 is, on a molar basis, three to five times as effective as T_4 in most systems and its effects have a more rapid onset and are less protracted.

Thyroid hormones have a wide variety of actions on many aspects of cell function; these will now be considered.

Calorigenesis

Thyroid hormones increase oxygen consumption and heat production by the organism as a whole and by certain tissues (see below). This effect is important in thermoregulation and in adaptation to environmental cold. Changes in heat production by the human subject can be used in the diagnosis of thyroid status by measurement of the basal metabolic rate (BMR). The effects occur after a latent period. Thus, after thyroidectomy, BMR declines progressively to between 30 to 50 per cent of the preoperative level over a period of thirty to forty days. Conversely, T_4 does not begin to increase BMR appreciably until twelve to twenty-four hours after administration, and to attain its maximal effect may take five to ten days. Most tissues increase their oxygen consumption and heat production in response to thyroid hormones, the main exceptions being brain, testes, spleen, uterus and anterior pituitary. In fact, the heat production and oxygen consumption of the anterior pituitary is reduced by T_4 and T_3, presumably as a result of the suppression of TSH secretion (p.106).

> The mechanism of the calorigenic action has been the subject of considerable debate. Since 90 per cent of the total body consumption of oxygen involves mitochondria, attention has focussed on the actions of T_4 and T_3 on these organelles. Early work suggested that the hormones uncoupled oxidation from oxidative phosphorylation such that catabolic energy would tend to appear as heat rather than energy-rich phosphate compounds. This explanation is not now generally accepted, since it has been shown that mitochondrial calorigenesis does not necessarily involve uncoupling; T_4 has now been shown to produce 'loose coupling', i.e. an acceleration of mitochondrial respiration without significant reduction in phosphorylation. The major part of this effect depends upon increased synthesis of protein, perhaps to provide mitochondrial electron carriers such as cytochrome C or oxidative enzymes such as cytochrome oxidase. This effect is delayed and could well account for the latent period before calorigenesis begins (see above): it can also be blocked by agents which block ribosomal transcription and translation. In addition to this effect, part of the action of T_4 and T_3 on heat production can be attributed to the 'permissive' effect they exert on the weak calorigenic action of other hormones such as the catecholamines, insulin, glucagon, growth hormone and glucocorticoids; in the hypothyroid individual the calorigenic effects of the other hormones are reduced or absent, whereas they are exaggerated in the hyperthyroid state. One further aspect of the calorigenic action of T_4 and T_3 may be the heat production which results from the stimulation of the sodium pump in cell membranes; between 20 and 50 per cent of the resting heat production is associated with the sodium pump and T_4 and T_3 can be shown to promote activity in the system.

Effects on carbohydrate and fat metabolism

Thyroid hormones have a number of actions on carbohydrate metabolism which mostly tend to increase glucose mobilization and plasma glucose concentrations (catabolic actions). Such actions include (a) stimulation of hepatic glycogenolysis, (b) stimulation of intestinal absorption of glucose, (c) potentiation of the glycogenolytic actions of other hormones such as adrenaline, and (d) stimulation of insulin breakdown. However, some other effects, including promotion of the entry of glucose into tissues such as muscle and adipose tissue, serve to potentiate the hypoglycaemic actions of insulin, as does the increased hepatic glycogenesis produced by *small* doses of T_4 (larger doses cause glycogenolysis).

Thyroid hormones affect most aspects of lipid metabolism and, as for carbohydrate discussed above, the net effect is usually catabolic, although some anabolic actions are present, particularly at low hormone concentrations.

Thyroxine and T_3 exert a powerful lipolytic action on fat stores, both as a direct effect and through potentiation of other lipolytic agents such as adrenaline, growth hormone, glycocorticoids and glucagon. There is also increased oxidation of the free fatty acids (FFA) released which contributes toward the calorigenic effect. Incorporation of some of the FFA into triglycerides in the liver is also stimulated. One of the very important actions of T_4 and T_3 is to lower plasma cholesterol. The major effect here is to stimulate oxidative processes such as bile acid formation in the liver and consequently faecal excretion of cholesterol derivatives, but some depletion of plasma cholesterol also results from stimulated steroid synthesis in the adrenal cortex (p.117) and gonads.

Effects on protein metabolism

Thyroid hormones stimulate the synthesis of specific proteins involved in calorigenesis (see above) but, in addition, small amounts of T_4 appear to be necessary for the maintenance of normal rates of protein synthesis in general: this effect probably results from stimulation of phosphorylation and the processes of translation and transcription (p.98). In support of this suggestion is the fact that protein synthesis is severely depressed in the hypothyroid state but can be returned to normal, after a latent period of two to three days, by treatment with *small* doses of T_4. This anabolic effect of T_4 and T_3 when present in low or physiological amounts, dramatically changes to a marked catabolic effect when the hormones are present in excess. Protein breakdown associated with thyroid overactivity is particularly marked in muscle, where the effect may be so severe as to cause muscular weakness (thyrotoxic myopathy). This protein catabolism results in an elevation in plasma amino acid concentrations and increased creatine excretion (creatinuria). If the increased catabolism cannot be matched by a corresponding increase in dietary protein intake, there is breakdown of body protein stores and loss of weight ensues.

One further aspect of protein metabolism relates to the subcutaneous deposition of mucoprotein associated with thyroid deficiency. Since this material is osmotically active, it sequesters water in the subcutaneous spaces and produces characteristic soft swellings (myxoedema). The mucoprotein can be dispersed by administration of thyroid hormone and the associated fluid is lost in the urine.

Effects on skeletal growth and development

In man there appears to be little, if any, transfer of maternal T_4 or T_3 to the embryo and fetus. During very early embryonic development, before the thyroid functions, growth seems to depend solely upon genetic factors, but once the fetal thyroid becomes functional, at ten to eleven weeks gestation, T_4 and T_3 become essential for the normal *differentiation* and *maturation* of fetal tissues, although lack of these hormones does not result in a significant reduction in fetal *growth*. Thus, human cretins are essentially normal in terms of birth weight, but have obvious deficiencies in skeletal and cerebral maturation.

Postnatally, thyroid hypofunction results in a severe depression of skeletal growth and of the development of almost all organ systems. Bone growth in hypothyroid infants is much retarded and dwarfism results, associated with the retention of infantile skeletal characteristics such as disproportionately short lower segment of the body and a broad, flat nose. The slow growth of bone is accompanied by delayed appearance and ossification of the epiphyses: dental development is also delayed. Replacement therapy can largely restore normal skeletal development and, if instituted early enough, can allow the patient to attain normal stature: this is not possible if thyroid deficiency persists to puberty. The optimal amount of thyroid hormones necessary for normal skeletal growth falls within a narrow range, for if too much T_4 is given to hypothyroid dwarfs the catabolic actions of the hormone predominate and the desired increase in growth and development does not take place. Excessive thyroid hormone availability during development usually produces some increase in stature, although the effect is not marked. Conversely, in certain individuals, premature closing of the epiphyses may stunt growth: this emphasizes once more the delicate hormonal balance required for growth.

Effects on the central nervous system

Adequate thyroid hormone during the late fetal and early postnatal period is vital to normal development of the CNS: thyroid deficiency at this time results in irreversible mental retardation (cretinism). However, if an early diagnosis can be made and replacement therapy instituted within three weeks of birth, almost all the neural consequences of thyroid deficiency can be forestalled. Why thyroid hormones are essential during the immediately postnatal period remains unclear, although a number of mechanisms may be involved. Thus, in the absence of these hormones, myelination of nerve fibre tracts is defective, there is a decrease in the size and number of neurones in the cerebral cortices, and the blood supply to the brain is reduced. Effects of deficiency or excess of thyroid hormones on nervous function in the adult will be discussed below.

Effects on the cardiovascular system

Thyroid hormones affect the cardiovascular system both directly and indirectly via their potentiating action on the effects of the catecholamines. In general the effects resemble those of activation of the sympathetic nervous system.

Effects of deficiency and excess of thyroid hormone

Many of the consequences of either a deficiency (hypothyroid) or an excess (hyperthyroid) of T_4 and T_3 can be predicted on the basis of the foregoing general description of the actions of these hormones. Consequently, for convenience these are summarized in Table 8.3

Table 8.3   Effects of thyroid deficiency and excess in relation to actions discussed in text

	Hypothyroid	Hyperthyroid
1. Calorigenesis	Low BMR; cold sensitivity	High BMR; heat sensitivity
2. Carbohydrate and lipid metabolism	Impaired intestinal glucose absorption; high plasma cholesterol	Enhanced intestinal glucose absorption; low plasma cholesterol
3. Protein metabolism	Decreased protein synthesis; myxoedema	Increased protein catabolism → negative nitrogen balance
4. Growth	Deficient growth at certain ages	
5. Effects on CNS	Cretinism if perinatal deficiency; sluggish mentation	Restless, overanxiety, irritable
6. Cardiovascular system	Decreased cardiac output and heart rate; increased circulation time	Increased cardiac output and heart rate; decreased circulation time

Causes of thyroid deficiency

Hypothyroidism is the term used to describe the condition where insufficient thyroid hormone is secreted: the older term 'myxoedema' is now used to describe specifically the subcutaneous mucoprotein deposition and associated fluid retention.

Hypothyroidism may result from the congenital deficiency or total absence of thyroid tissue in the infant, while in the adult it results if severe thyroid damage is caused surgically, by radio-iodine or by x-ray therapy. Thyroid function can also be reduced by antithyroid drugs, auto-immune disease (e.g. Hashimoto's disease) or chronic iodine deficiency (Daggett: *Clinical Endocrinology*, Chapter 4). Finally, inadequate activity by an otherwise healthy thyroid can result if TSH secretion is impaired, either by disease of the anterior pituitary itself or by hypothalamic malfunction. If the deficiency originates in the thyroid itself it will not respond to TSH. If function can be restored by TSH but not TRH the site of failure is probably the anterior pituitary, whereas if TRH is effective, hypothalamic deficiency must be suspected. Although TSH and TRH can be valuable to diagnosis, as described above, T_4 and sometimes T_3 are, by virtue of their much longer half-lives, the hormones used to treat hypothyroidism itself.

Causes of excessive thyroid activity

Hyperthyroidism or thyrotoxicosis are terms used to describe the condition where thyroid secretion is abnormally high: this is almost always the direct consequence of primary thyroid overactivity.

Enlargement of the thyroid associated with hyperfunction (toxic goitre) can produce a wide spectrum of symptoms and has given rise to an equally diffuse nomenclature. Graves' disease is the commonest in which goitre is associated with thyrotoxicosis and exophthalmos (forward displacement of the eyeball (Daggett: *Clinical Endocrinology*, Chapter 4). The eyeball is displaced by the growth of a small pad of fat in the tissue behind the globe of the eye. This process is not affected by either TSH or TSI (see below) and is held by some to be due to a specific 'exophthalmos-producing substance' (EPS) of pituitary origin. However, exophthalmos has been recently shown to occur even after hypophysectomy and it is now thought that the agent responsible is an immunoglobulin.

Immunoglobulins and thyroid stimulation

While attempting unsuccessfully to demonstrate elevated TSH levels in the blood of patients with Graves' disease, Adams and Purves, in 1956, found that the blood often contained another factor with a much more protracted thyroid-stimulating action: this was named the long-acting thyroid stimulator (LATS). It is now known that LATS is one of a group of IgG immunoglobulins which affect the thyroid, termed thyroid-stimulating immunoglobulins (TSI), or thyroid-stimulating antibodies (TSAb). There is much still to be learned of the part played by TSAb in human thyroid disease. They are believed to be produced in response to undefined stimuli by thymus-dependent lymphocytes in certain individuals with a genetic predisposition and may act as antibodies against thyroid antigens. The specific role of LATS in the aetiology of Graves' disease remains uncertain, for LATS is found in the serum of less than 80 per cent of sufferers and the amount present often does not correlate with the severity of the disease (Daggett: *Clinical Endocrinology*, Chapter 4). In LATS-negative patients with hyperthyroid disease, a second immunoglobulin may be present which acts to prevent the inactivation of LATS by thyroid protein: this second IgG has been called 'LATS protector'.

The actions of LATS on the thyroid are similar to those of TSH in that both increase adenyl cyclase activity; but, while the effects of TSH are rapid and transient, those of LATS are progressive and prolonged. Thyroid hormones suppress TSH production by negative feedback at the pituitary level, but do not effect LATS production: hence, in toxic goitre, LATS is elevated while TSH levels are low.

Excessive thyroid hormone secretion is also found in benign and, more rarely, malignant tumours of the follicular cells.

Goitre

Goitre is the general term used to describe swelling of the thyroid gland; when such swellings result in excess hormone secretion they are termed 'toxic goitres' (see above). The other principal category of goitre is the simple or 'nontoxic' goitre which is associated with normal (euthyroid) hormone secretion and represents essentially a compensatory hypertrophy of the gland in response to circumstances where its hormone production mechanism has been impaired. For example, dietary iodine deficiency is associated with goitre: such a goitre is said to be 'endemic' if it occurs within a restricted geographical area where natural iodine supplies are low (e.g. 'Derbyshire neck', and the 'goitre belt' in the central part of the USA) and 'sporadic' when it occurs elsewhere. Goitre can also result from the ingestion of chemicals which interfere with thyroid function, such as antithyroid drugs and goitrogens in the diet (Daggett: *Clinical Endocrinology*, Chapter 4). The latter are found in vegetables such as cabbage and turnips (Brassicaceae), although, on a normal mixed diet, and particularly when the vegetables are cooked, only trivial amounts of the active principle, **goitrin**, are absorbed. Other varieties of simple goitre may be due to the increased thyroid hormone requirement at puberty or during pregnancy or lactation. It may also be found as a result of congenital deficiencies in thyroid enzyme systems (goitrous cretinism).

Control of the secretion of thyroxine (T₄) and tri-iodothyronine (T₃)

The secretions of the thyroid gland, like those of other endocrine glands, are closely regulated. However, regulation is particularly important in the case of the thyroid in view of the delayed and protracted mode of action of T_4 and T_3. To some extent, acute fluctuation in the availability of these hormones to tissues is prevented by both the 'reservoir' of hormone bound to plasma proteins and by the large store of hormone retained in the form of thyroglobulin within the gland itself. Nevertheless, the rate of synthesis of T_4 and T_3 is subject to close control, both by intrathyroidal mechanisms serving to stabilize the size of the pool of stored hormone and by the action of TSH, which also dictates the rate of release of stored hormone into the circulation. Outside the thyroid itself, TSH secretion is promoted by TRH from the hypothalamus but inhibited by a negative feedback of T_4 and T_3 on the pituitary. In turn, TRH secretion is influenced by neural factors and by relatively undefined feedback actions of thyroid hormones and TSH. The overall arrangement of the hypothalamic-pituitary-thyroid axis is shown in Fig. 8.4. We shall now analyse the properties of this system: first, by considering each process in turn, as numbered in Fig. 8.4, and secondly, by attempting an overview of how these processes and other factors interact in the

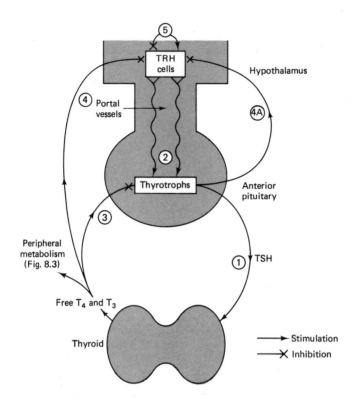

Fig. 8.4 An overall view of the factors regulating thyroid secretion (see text). T_4 = thyroxine; TSH = thyroid-stimulating hormone; TRH = thyrotrophin-releasing hormone.

regulation of thyroid activity. First, however, it is appropriate to point out that more is known about the control of thyroid secretion than about that from any other gland controlled by the adenohypophysis. Moreover, studies of thyroid control have, until very recently, been far in advance of those elsewhere. The reason for this is quite simply that until the development of modern specific analytical techniques, and in particular radio-immunoassay, it was technically impossible to measure accurately and specifically peptide hormones in blood. In consequence, all quantitative studies of adenohypophyseal activity relied upon some type of biological assay to determine hormone concentrations. All these, with the exception of the TSH assay described below, were cumbersome, insensitive and relatively inaccurate.

The fact that T_4 and T_3 contain iodine atoms allows them to be labelled with an isotope such as ^{131}I or ^{125}I. This has greatly facilitated investigation of all aspects of thyroid function and, in particular, studies of the control of thyroid secretion. Perhaps the most widely used and intrinsically important technique is that described in Fig. 8.5. Almost all the general principles of the interactions of the components of the hypothalamo-pituitary-thyroid axis shown in Fig. 8.4 were first demonstrated using this technique, although of

(a) Rabbit on low-iodine diet (Day-2)

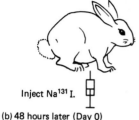

Inject Na^{131}I.

During the 48 hours after the Na^{131}I is injected most ^{131}I enters the thyroid and is incorporated into ^{131}I T$_4$ and ^{131}I T$_3$. The remaining ^{131}I which escapes the thyroid iodide trap is either lost in the urine or enters stable combination with non-thyroidal tissues.

(b) 48 hours later (Day 0)
Thiocyanate injection blocks iodide trap

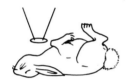

Injection of thiocyanate prevents the re-uptake into the thyroid of any ^{131}I from deiodination of ^{131}I T$_4$ subsequently secreted.

The neck radioactivity gives a measure of the store of labelled T$_4$ when corrected for non-specific ^{131}I binding by subtracting the value for the control area of leg (tissue background)

Measure radioactivity over thyroid region and over control area of leg. (Tissue background.) Animal lightly anaesthetized.

(c)

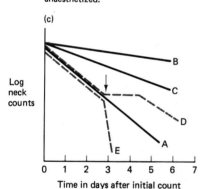

Log neck counts

Time in days after initial count

The neck radioactivity corrected for the tissue background and physical decay of the isotope is then recorded at intervals thereafter. If the results are plotted on semi-log graph paper, the exponential decrease in neck radioactivity appears as a straight line. The slope of this line gives a measure of the rate of release of T$_4$ and thus, indirectly, of endogenous TSH secretion.

The changes recorded with this technique under 5 circumstances are shown highly digrammatically in c); A normal; B hypophysectomy; C hypophysectomy plus intra-ocular transplant; D normal with T$_4$ injection at arrow; E normal with TSH injection at arrow.

Fig. 8.5 Diagram to illustrate the classical method of assessing T$_4$ and TSH by measuring neck radioactivity after Na^{131}I administration.

course modern assay methods which allow *direct* measurement of hormones are now employed for thyroid work and have also permitted detailed studies on other endocrine systems.

The hypothalamo-pituitary-thyroid axis (text numbers correspond with those in Fig. 8.4)

1. *The action of TSH on the thyroid*
It has long been known that hypophysectomy leads to thyroid atrophy and decreased function and that administration of pituitary extract will restore

thyroid activity. The hormone concerned is the glycoprotein TSH (p.79). It is secreted by the pituitary thyrotrophs and can be shown to influence virtually every aspect of thyroid function, including the promotion within a matter of minutes of iodide uptake and synthesis and release of T_4 and T_3 and, after a longer delay, increase in thyroid mass. Thyroid-stimulating hormone exerts its effects after binding to the surface of thyroid cells and activating adenyl cyclase. The action of cAMP is mediated via a protein kinase. It is unusual in that Ca^{2+} does not seem to be required, but there is some recent evidence to implicate prostaglandins in the process.

2. *The action of TRH on TSH*

Cold has long been known to promote T_4 secretion and, as this stimulus is ineffective in hypophysectomized animals, the effect must involve TSH release. Moreover, since cold has no action on T_4 secretion if the pituitary stalk is sectioned or if the pituitary is transplanted to a remote site, it follows that the pathway also includes pituitary stimulation by a chemical released into the portal vessels in the hypothalamus: this substance is TRH and has been discussed elsewhere (p.73). Electrical stimulation over a relatively large area of the anterior hypothalamus will increase TSH secretion and is associated with the appearance of TRH in portal blood. It seems that TRH is secreted continuously and this 'tonic' background of TRH is necessary for normal TSH release (Daggett: *Clinical Endocrinology*, Chapter 5). However, rapid neurally mediated changes in TRH secretion can be superimposed upon the background secretion (see p.108), particularly since TRH has a very short biological half-life (approximately four minutes). The importance of TRH to normal TSH release is shown in Fig. 8.5c, which illustrates the decrease in endogenous T_4 release (and hence TSH release) when the pituitary is transplanted to the eye. However, it should be noted that the decrease is less than that following hypophysectomy, indicating that TSH release is not *totally* dependent upon TRH (Fig. 8.5b).

The TRH affects the thyrotrophs after attachment to the cell membrane by activation of adenyl cyclase and promotes both synthesis and secretion of TSH.

3. *Thyroid hormone feedback at the pituitary level*

It is well established that T_4 depresses TSH secretion (Fig. 8.6) and, conversely, that thyroidectomy, by removing this negative feedback, results in a dramatic rise in circulating TSH and the appearance in the pituitary of many mucoprotein-containing 'thyroidectomy' cells presumed to be the source of the extra TSH. The inverse curvilinear relation between free T_4 and TSH is illustrated in Fig. 8.6. Such evidence does not, however, indicate whether the site of feedback is at the pituitary level or within the brain. Early work appeared to show unequivocally that T_4 injected into the pituitary suppressed TSH, whereas intrahypothalamic injection was without effect. Moreover, T_4 will suppress and thyroidectomy will enhance the residual TSH secretion by a pituitary transplanted to the anterior chamber of the eye.

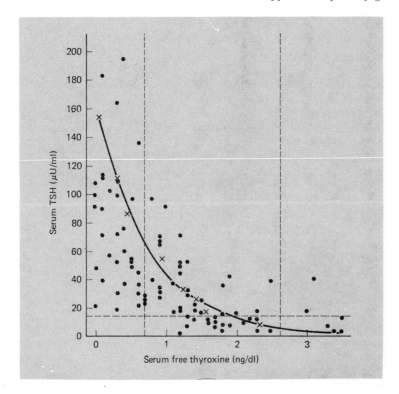

Fig. 8.6 Relation between serum TSH and serum-free T_4 in patients with myxoedema given various doses of L-thyroxine. Horizontal dashed line indicates normal upper limit for TSH and vertical dashed limits enclose normal range for T_4. Solid curved line is regression line based on the mean values at each dose of T_4. (From Colton G. E., Gorman, C. H. and Mayberry, W. E. (1971). *New England Journal of Medicine* **185**, 529.)

4. *Thyroid hormone feedback at the hypothalamic level*
The questions of whether and how thyroid hormones effect TRH synthesis and release remain unresolved. Some workers claim that T_4 injected into the hypothalamus inhibits TRH (negative feedback), but the amounts used were large and the possibility of carriage of T_4 down the portal vessels to the pituitary cannot be excluded. On the other hand, it has been claimed that T_4 promotes the synthesis of TRH by hypothalamic tissue *in vitro* (positive feedback). Whatever may eventually transpire to be the true situation, it is clear that the most important and *over-riding* feedback effect is the direct suppression of TSH by thyroid hormones at pituitary level. Claims for a short-loop negative feedback of TSH on TRH (see pathway in 4a in Fig. 8.4) are now largely discounted.

5. *The control of TRH secretion*
The neural stimulus for the tonic release of TRH necessary to normal TSH

secretion originates within the hypothalamus itself, since isolating the hypothalamus totally from the rest of the brain does not impair the basal function of the pituitary-thyroid axis. More precise localized destruction within the hypothalamus indicates that the paraventricular, ventromedial and arcuate nuclei are particularly involved and correlates well with the results of electrical stimulation.

Cold promotes an immediate and short-lived (acute) surge of TSH as a result of stimulation of TRH release. In rats the effect is over within sixty minutes and appears to be a simple neuroendocrine reflex from peripheral cold receptors. Similar responses occur in the human infant, but little, if any, effect has been demonstrated in adults. The responses to chronic cold are less well established and so far there have been no convincing demonstrations of a maintained increase in thyroid secretion in man.

Stress results in inhibition of TSH secretion through a variety of mechanisms. The immediate and rapid fall in TSH must represent a neurally mediated pathway and, despite early claims for an inhibiting factor, seem now due to a sudden fall in TRH secretion. Thereafter, other hormones released during stress, particularly the glucocorticoids, probably exert a secondary suppressive action on pituitary TSH production. This suppressive action of glucocorticoids may explain the diurnal pattern of TSH secretion which is out of phase with the diurnal variation in glucocorticoid secretion.

Monoaminergic neurones seem to be implicated in the control of TRH release (see Fig. 7.5); thus, noradrenaline stimulates and serotonin inhibits the process.

The sympathetic nervous system and thyroid secretion

Much recent attention has been directed toward the role of the sympathetic innervation to the thyroid. It seems that activity in these nerves, or the presence of catecholamines in blood, can directly stimulate thyroid secretion. The responsiveness of the thyroid to such stimulation depends to a large extent upon the TSH levels and, in any event, sympathetic effects are probably quantitatively insignificant relative to TSH. However, one interesting qualitative effect of sympathetic influences supported by preliminary evidence, is that they modulate the action of TSH in favour of the production of more T_3 in relation to T_4.

Thyroid control: a recapitulation

The level of free thyroid hormone in blood is buffered by the relatively huge reservoir of protein-bound hormone, but is still regulated with exquisite sensitivity. The primary short-term regulation devolves upon the negative feedback loop between thyroid hormone and the thyrotroph (see pathways 1 and 3 in Fig. 8.4). However, the set-point for the feedback is determined by the tonic level of TRH secreted by the hypothalamus (see pathway 2 in Fig. 8.4). Thus, acute regulation of secretion depends upon the interplay of the stimulating effects of TRH and the inhibiting effects of thyroid hormones. A neurally promoted increase in TRH in response to, for example, cold, results in a rapid increase in TSH secretion, while TSH secretion can be suppressed, after a short delay, by thyroid hormones, which can also prevent or reduce

TRH-mediated stimulation of TSH. Tonic TRH secretion sufficient to maintain near-normal pituitary-thyroid function requires the integrity of only the medial basal hypothalmus, but changes in TRH in response to cold, stress etc. require other regions of the brain. Feedback effects of thyroid hormones or TSH on the hypothalamus have been claimed (see pathways 4 and 4a in Fig. 8.4) and may play a role in the long-term regulation of thyroid function, but do not contribute significantly in the short term.

The sympathetic nervous system may influence thyroid secretion by decreasing the ratio of $T_4:T_3$ produced and much still remains to be resolved about the physiological importance of T_3 in the control of thyroid activity.

Calcitonin (CT)

Calcitonin (CT, previously called thyrocalcitonin) is a peptide hormone which lowers blood calcium concentration and increases urinary phosphate excretion: it acts as a physiological antagonist to parathormone (Chapter 2) but appears to play a relatively minor role in calcium homeostasis in adult man (Chapter 12).

Anatomy and microstructure

Calcitonin is secreted by the C cells of the mammalian thyroid. In fish, reptiles, amphibia and birds the C cells are grouped in the ultimobranchial bodies: these are derived from neural crest material and arise from the last branchial pouch. In mammals, the ultimobranchial bodies fuse with the thyroid during early embryogenesis and thus the C cells have become incorporated within the thyroid gland.

The C cells, often called parafollicular cells, are difficult to identify in conventional histological preparations, but are epithelial in appearance and situated in the stroma between the thyroid follicles: prominent granules within the cytoplasm are presumed to contain CT.

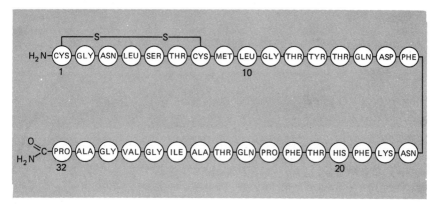

Fig. 8.7 Structure of human calcitonin.

Chemistry and metabolism of calcitonin

Human CT consists of a single polypeptide chain of 32 amino acids (Fig. 8.7), it has a molecular weight of 3421. There are considerable species differences in the amino acid sequence, but 7 of the 9 N-terminal amino acids are identical in all species studied, which suggests strongly that the biological activity is associated with this part of the molecule.

Calcitonin distributes throughout the extracellular fluid and has a disappearance rate too rapid to be explained by glomerular filtration. Recent studies suggest that it can be degraded within the liver and kidney: the half-life is probably of the order of thirty minutes.

Actions of calcitonin

The principal action of CT is to reduce blood calcium concentration by inhibiting the resorption of bone mineral. In addition, it has been claimed that CT may increase the urinary excretion of calcium and phosphate and may influence intestinal absorption of calcium. There is considerable evidence to indicate that CT is of much greater physiological importance in young animals than in adults. Figure 8.8 demonstrates the dramatic decline in the effectiveness of CT with respect to age in the rat.

Effect on bone

Much evidence is now available to indicate that CT inhibits the movement of calcium from bone mineral to the blood, leading to a depression of bone resorption: this action directly opposes the action of PTH on bone. Calcitonin appears to work principally on the cells within bone and reduces both osteocytic and osteoclastic activity.

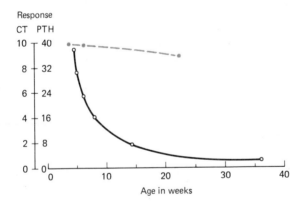

Fig. 8.8 Effect of age on relative responsiveness of rats to PTH (•–•) and CT (o–o). The marked decline in response to CT with age reflects the decreasing rate of skeletal remodelling. (From Copp, D. H. (1969). *Annual Review of Pharmacology* **9**, 327.)

Effect on the kidney

It has been claimed that CT increases the urinary excretion of both calcium and phosphate, although the latter effect appears to require the presence of PTH. The amounts of CT necessary to produce significant renal effects are almost certainly unphysiologically high, so it is generally accepted that CT probably has little, if any, direct effect on the kidney under normal circumstances.

Effect on the intestine

In vitro experiments appear to show that CT depresses calcium absorption from the intestine. Experiments on intact animals or human subjects have shown, in contrast, that CT usually enhances calcium absorption, probably indirectly as a result of the PTH released in response to the hypocalcaemia induced by CT. On balance, it is likely that the *direct* effect of CT on intestinal calcium absorption is not significant.

Effect of deficiency

The role of CT in normal calcium homeostatis in adult man is still unclear (see Chapter 12). It is likely that small amounts of CT are secreted continuously at normal blood calcium levels. *However, there are no obvious manifestations of CT deficiency in totally thyroidectomized patients treated only with thyroxine.*

Effect of excess

Medullary carcinoma of the thyroid, a relatively rare form of thyroid malignancy, comprises neoplasia of the C cells and results in excess production of CT. Despite the elevated blood level of CT, there are rarely, if ever, significant disturbances in calcium metabolism, probably since there is usually a compensating increase in PTH secretion which tends to counteract the potential effects of excess CT (Daggett: *Clinical Endocrinology*, Chapter 7). Administration of CT has been shown to have some value in the treatment of Paget's disease, a condition in which excessive reabsorption of bone takes place.

Control of calcitonin secretion

Like that of PTH, the secretion of CT appears to depend solely upon the concentration of ionized calcium in the blood. Elevation of blood calcium promotes CT secretion, whereas a fall in blood calcium depresses its release. It should be noted, however, that at the present time it is extremely difficult to obtain an accurate measurement of CT levels in the blood of normal subjects. The role of CT in calcium metabolism and its interactions with PTH and vitamin D will be discussed further in Chapter 12.

Further reading

Daggett, Peter (1981). *Clinical Endocrinology*. Edward Arnold, London.

Greep, R. O. and Astwood, E. B. (1974). Endocrinology: Handbook of Physiology, Vol. III. *Thyroid*. American Physiological Society, Washington.

Werner, S. C. and Ingbar, S. H. (Eds.) (1971). *The Thyroid, a Fundamental and Clinical Text*, 3rd edn. Harper and Row, New York.

Werner, S. C. and Ingbar, S. H. (Eds.) (1978). *The Thyroid*, 4th edn. Harper and Row, New York.

9

The adrenal cortex

The adrenal cortex completely envelopes the medulla but, in spite of this intimate anatomical relationship, the two endocrine tissues are quite distinct entities, having separate embryological origins and secreting different types of hormone. The most important feature that the adrenal cortex and medulla have in common is the fact that both respond to a wide variety of so-called 'stresses'.

The adrenal cortex comprises three morphologically distinct regions, each of which produces a different type of steroid hormone. The outmost region (**zona glomerulosa**) secretes aldosterone and thereby controls sodium reabsorption in the renal tubules and elsewhere. The **zona reticularis** encircles the medulla and synthesizes both oestrogens and androgens. The latter are responsible for the virilism which occurs sometimes in women with adrenal tumours, but their function, if any, under normal physiological conditions is unknown. The **zona fasciculata** occupies an intermediary position between the other two regions and produces the glucocorticoids, cortisol and corticosterone, which have widespread effects on carbohydrate, fat and protein metabolism.

Anatomy and microstructure

The adrenal cortex develops from cells of the coelomic mesoderm, near the anterior pole of the mesonephros, which start to proliferate in the human fetus at the 8–10 mm stage. It is thought that the original masses develop into the fetal adrenal cortex in the human and that the permanent cortex arises from a later proliferation of cells at or near the original site which come to surround the first population.

> The adrenal medulla arises from ectodermal cells which migrate from the neural crests to penetrate the primordial adrenal nodule and come to occupy the central region (see Chapter 3).

The gland is contained within a well-defined capsule of connective tissue, under which the cells of the zona glomerulosa are arranged in small clusters and arcades of parenchymatous cells closely associated with numerous capillaries. The arcades of the zona glomerulosa are continuous with the columns of polyhedral cells which comprise the zona fasciculata. These columns are fairly regularly aligned at right angles to the surface and are surrounded by straight capillaries running in the same direction. These cells are larger than those of the glomerulosa and are normally packed with fat droplets, but special staining techniques are required to visualize these as they are lost during treatment with organic solvents. Deeply, the zona fasciculata merges gradually into the zona reticularis in which the cells are disposed in an anastomosing network. Many of these cells have dark nuclei and acidophilic cytoplasm which suggests that they may be degenerating.

Electron micrographs of adrenal cortical parenchyma confirm the presence of large numbers of fat droplets and reveal two other distinctive features of these cells: 1) an abundance of smooth endoplasmic reticulum and a relative lack of rough endoplasmic reticulum; 2) mitochondria in which the inner membrane forms finger-like invaginations, or even vesicles, instead of the lamellae that are so typical of mitochondria in other tissues.

These ultrastructural features can be modified experimentally by exposing animals to conditions which influence adrenal secretory activity and therefore seem to be related to the rate of hormone production. A high-sodium diet, which inhibits release of aldosterone, causes an increase in the population of lipid droplets in the zona glomerulosa, together with a reduction in smooth endoplasmic reticulum and vesiculated mitochondria: the converse is observed following sodium depletion. In the zona fasciculata, hypophysectomy reduces the amount of smooth endoplasmic reticulum and the number of mitochondria and the latter lose their vesicles; these changes are reversed by the administration of adrenocorticotrophin (ACTH). The structural changes are presumably related to changes in the rates of various synthetic reactions in the endoplasmic reticulum and mitochondria and the amounts of lipid, cholesterol and/or steroid stored in the fat droplets (see Fig. 9.2).

Chemistry and metabolism of hormones

Structure

All the adrenal cortical hormones are steroids derived initially from cholesterol, the essential nucleus of which (cyclopentanoperhydrophenanthrene nucleus; Fig. 9.1a) is preserved through all the various biosynthetic steps. Steroid hormones are produced by the adrenal cortex, the testis and the ovary, all of which develop from the same embryonic tissue (the mesoderm of the urogenital ridge) and the initial biosynthetic steps in the production of all steroid hormones are the same. The end products fall into two main categories: those with a two-carbon side chain attached at C17, which are referred to as C21 steroids (Fig. 9.1b) and those with either an $= 0$ or $-OH$ group at C17, which are termed C19 steroids (Fig. 9.1c). The C19 steroids possess androgenic activity but removal of a further carbon atom results in C18 compounds with oestrogenic properties. The C21 steroids possess both mineralocorticoid and glucocorticoid activity and the further small differences in structure between them determines which of these predominates. The differences are very pronounced, however, and the naturally occurring mineralocorticoid, aldosterone, possesses some 2000 times

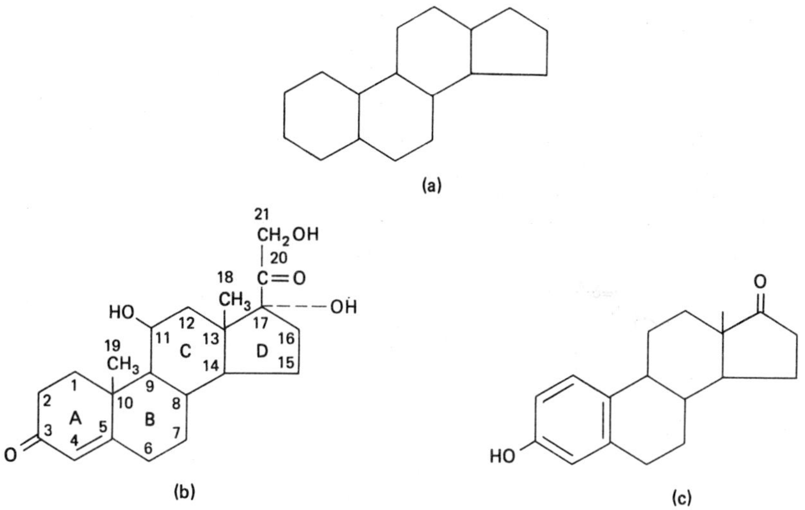

Fig. 9.1 (a) The cyclopentanoperhydrophenanthrene nucleus. (b) A C21 steroid—cortisol. (c) A C18 steroid—oestrone.

the mineralocorticoid activity of the glucocorticoids, cortisol and corticosterone. Thus, in the amounts in which it is secreted in the body, it exerts highly effective control over sodium excretion without any significant glucocorticoid effect.

The double bonds between C4 and C5 and the ketone group at C3 are both indispensible to normal adrenocorticoid activity. An = 0 or – OH group at C11 is necessary for significant glucocorticoid, but not mineralocorticoid, activity, and glucocorticoid activity is further enhanced by the presence of an – OH group at C17. The presence of an = 0 or an – OH group at C21 is a prerequisite for a significant mineralocorticoid activity. The fact that the effects of these steroids can be modified so substantially by comparatively small variations in molecular structure has led to the production of a wide range of synthetic steroids for therapeutic purposes. Many of these are fluorinated at the 9-α position (triamcinolone, dexamethasone, fludrocortisone) as this greatly enhances the biological potency.

Biosynthesis

Some of the steps involved in the synthesis of cortisol and corticosterone in the zona fasciculata are shown diagrammatically in Fig. 9.2a and identified by number in the following description.

The scheme illustrated in the diagram complies with the evidence at present available regarding the localization of the various enzyme reactions within the cell. However, it is at best a simplified scheme and may well need to be modified in the light of further information. So far as we can tell at present, all the synthetic enzymes are localized within either the smooth endoplasmic reticulum or the mitochondria and none is to be found in the fat droplets which represent a very rich store of cholesterol.

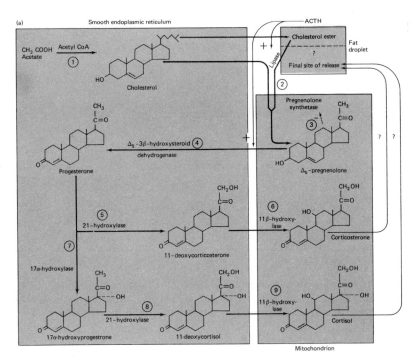

Fig. 9.2 Diagram to illustrate the synthesis of (**a**) glucocorticoid hormones, (**b**) mineralocorticoid hormones, and (**c**) androgens (see text).

It is supposed that certain steps in the process of steroidogenesis depend upon passage of substrate from the endoplasmic reticulum to the mitochondria or vice versa; this must occur very rapidly to account for the high rates of secretion which are known to occur, since only trivial amounts of these hormones are actually stored in the gland. In this connection it may be relevant that electron micrographs show frequent close relationships between smooth endoplasmic reticulum and fat droplets and between mitochondria and fat droplets. Perhaps the fat droplet represents the intracellular path along which the substrates pass between one synthetic site and the other.

Cholesterol is synthesized from acetate in the presence of acetyl CoA in the smooth endoplasmic reticulum (1) and is also taken up from the blood. Much is stored in the form of a cholesterol ester in the fat droplets and the rate at which cholesterol is released from this store by the action of a lipase (2) is believed to be a rate-limiting step in the biosynthesis of the glucocorticoids and to be controlled by ACTH (see below). In the mitochondria, free cholesterol is converted to $\triangle^5$ pregnenolone by pregnenolone synthetase which cleaves the side chain at C18 (3). This reaction is also thought to be rate limiting as the enzyme is susceptible to 'product inhibition'; it is suggested that this may be overcome in the presence of ACTH by increased permeability of the mitochondrial membrane to pregnenolone. In the smooth endoplasmic reticulum, pregnenolone is converted to progesterone by $\triangle^5$-3β-hydroxy-steroid dehydrogenase (4) which is then hydroxylated either at C21 (5) or C17 (7). The C21 hydroxylated derivative (11β-deoxycorticosterone) is finally hydroxylated at C11 in the mitochondria to corticosterone (6). The 17α-hydroxylation of progesterone in the smooth endoplasmic reticulum (7) leads to the production of cortisol by subsequent hydroxylations identical with those for corticosterone (8 and 9). Thus the activity of the enzyme 17α-hydroxylase determines the proportion of the two steroids secreted: this varies from species to species. Rats and mice produce corticosterone almost exclusively, whereas primates, ruminants, cats and guinea-pigs secrete more cortisol than corticosterone.

In the zona glomerulosa, corticosterone is converted to aldosterone within the mitochondria (Fig. 9.2b) by successive hydroxylation and dehydrogenation at the C18 position (6_G, 7_G).

In the zona reticularis, pregnenolone is converted to 17α-hydroxy-pregnenolone by the direct action of 17α-hydroxylase in the smooth endoplasmic reticulum. The side chain at C17 is then cleaved to produce the C19 steroid, dehydroepiandrosterone, which is converted to androstenedione by dehydrogenation (Fig. 9.2c).

Adrenal steroid hormones are liberated as soon as they are synthesized and only trace amounts can be detected in the gland. Thus the rate of secretion is determined by the rate of production. In the zona fasciculata this is controlled exclusively by ACTH, which attaches to specific receptors on the surface of the cells and causes a rapid increase in glucocorticoid production. The mechanism whereby this is achieved is still not fully understood, but most workers believe that ACTH stimulates steroidogenesis by two separate, but closely integrated, effects on the cell: 1) there is an increase in the permeability of the membrane to certain ions; 2) adenyl cyclase is activated leading to the production of cAMP. Protein kinase, activated by cAMP (see Chapter 1) is thought to phosphorylate two separate proteins, one of which acts as a lipase and mobilizes cholesterol from its bound form in the fat droplets, while the other promotes the conversion of cholesterol to pregnenolone (Fig. 9.2**a**). Further steroidogenesis depends upon sequential hydroxylation reactions with a high requirement for reduced triphosphopyridine nucleotide (TPNH). This is provided, via the pentose phosphate pathway, from glucose entering the cell, also in response to ACTH stimulation; oxidative metabolism of glucose provides ATP necessary to maintain cAMP production.

> Maximum steroidogenesis in response to ACTH occurs when only a tiny fraction of the available receptors are engaged. This excess of receptors greatly enhances the sensitivity of the adrenal cortical cells to the hormone, in the same way as the sensitivity of the liver to glucagon is enhanced (see Chapter 4).

In addition to these immediate effects of ACTH, following its attachment to the receptor sites, it also exerts a pronounced trophic effect on the adrenal cortex. Adrenocorticotrophin is necessary for normal growth, development and maintenance of the adrenal cortex, which atrophies quite rapidly after removal of the pituitary, unless ACTH is administered. Adrenocorticotrophin also causes adrenal vasodilation leading to increased blood flow through the gland. This effect is entirely separate from the effect on steroidogenesis and persists when production of glucocorticoids has been blocked by metabolic inhibitors.

The regulation of aldosterone secretion is believed to be mediated by the renin-angiotensin system. ACTH and the plasma concentrations of Na^+ and K^+. Increasingly, it seems that the renin-angiotensin system is the primary control mechanism and angiotensin appears to act by mobilizing cAMP. ACTH stimulates release of aldosterone directly and also enhances aldosterone release in response to angiotensin.

Comparatively little is known about the mechanisms whereby the adrenal steroids are released. The most that can be said is that results of studies using the electron microscope suggest that the newly synthesized hormones may pass into the fat droplets prior to release by a process resembling exocytosis. Electron micrographs of adrenal cortex show that the membranes of these droplets become fused to the cell membrane and rupture at the point of contact.

In the circulation, both glucocorticoids and mineralocorticoids tend to bind with plasma proteins; cortisol and corticosterone combine mainly with an α-globulin, which has been designated **corticosteroid-binding globulin** (CBG) or **transcortin**, and with less affinity to albumin.

> The general consequences of protein binding are described in detail in Chapter 8 relating to the thyroid, because thyroxine is almost entirely bound to plasma protein and therefore provides by far the best example. Precisely the same considerations apply in the case of the glucocorticoids, except that about 10 per cent is present in the 'free' form and about 90 per cent is bound. Aldosterone is even more loosely bound and 30 to 50 per cent is normally 'free' in man, but the absolute amounts of aldosterone in the plasma are minute by comparison with total glucocorticoid concentration (Table 9.1).
>
> Hormone which is bound to plasma protein is physiologically inert and is protected from loss by renal filtration or metabolic degradation in the tissues.

Table 9.1 Characteristics of circulating adrenal corticoids in man

	Total plasma concentration	Percentage bound	Half-life
Cortisol 0800 hours	140–700 nmol/l (5–25 µg/dl)		
2400 hours	Less than 140 nmol/l (less than 5 µg/dl)	Approx. 90	50–90 minutes
Corticosterone	Approx. 35 nmol/l (1 µg/dl)		
Aldosterone (mean ± SEM)			
Recumbent	92 ± 75 pmol/l (3.4 ± 2.8 ng/dl)		
Ambulent	378 ± 169 pmol/l (14.3 ± 6.4 ng/dl)	Approx. 60	15–25 minutes

This is why aldosterone disappears from the circulation so much more rapidly than the glucocorticoids (Table 9.1). The bound form represents an inactive reservoir of steroid hormone which can be converted rapidly to the free, active form by dissociation in the plasma.

An important consequence of protein binding in the case of the adrenal corticoids is stabilization of the pool of free hormone, because the rates at which these steroids are released from the adrenal cortex are highly variable. Under resting conditions there is a pronounced circadian rhythm, maximum rates of secretion occurring around 06.00 hours, and the hormones are generally released in spurts in response to various specific stimuli, even though the stimulus may persist for prolonged periods. At low rates of secretion, the reservoir of bound hormone is steadily depleted, thereby maintaining an equilibrium between that which is free and that bound to or metabolized by peripheral tissues. At high rates of secretion this reservoir is replenished and the rise in total plasma steroid concentration can be accounted for largely by an increase in the fraction which is bound.

Metabolism and excretion

Glucocorticoids
The concentration of any hormone in the plasma is determined primarily by two processes—the rate of secretion and rate of removal.

The latter is most conveniently expressed as the hypothetical volume of plasma that is completely cleared of the hormone in unit time or the **metabolic clearance rate** (MCR). It can be measured by infusing radioactive hormone intravenously at constant rate until the labelled hormone achieves a constant concentration in the plasma when the rate of removal is equal to the rate of infusion.

At this equilibrium:

$$\text{MCR (litres/hour)} = \frac{\text{Rate of infusion } (\mu g/\text{hour})}{\text{Plasma concentration } (\mu g/\text{litre})}$$

The rate of secretion of endogenous hormone can then be estimated according to the equation:

$$\text{Plasma concentration } (\mu g/\text{litre}) = \frac{\text{Rate of secretion } (\mu g/\text{hour})}{\text{MCR (litres/hour)}}$$

The main technical problem which arises stems from the fact that metabolism of the hormone leads to the reappearance of nonspecific radioactivity in the plasma, for which it is often difficult to make appropriate correction. It is also important to realize that the MCR will vary with plasma concentration, unless the rate at which the hormone is lost depends entirely on concentration gradient and disappearance is strictly exponential.

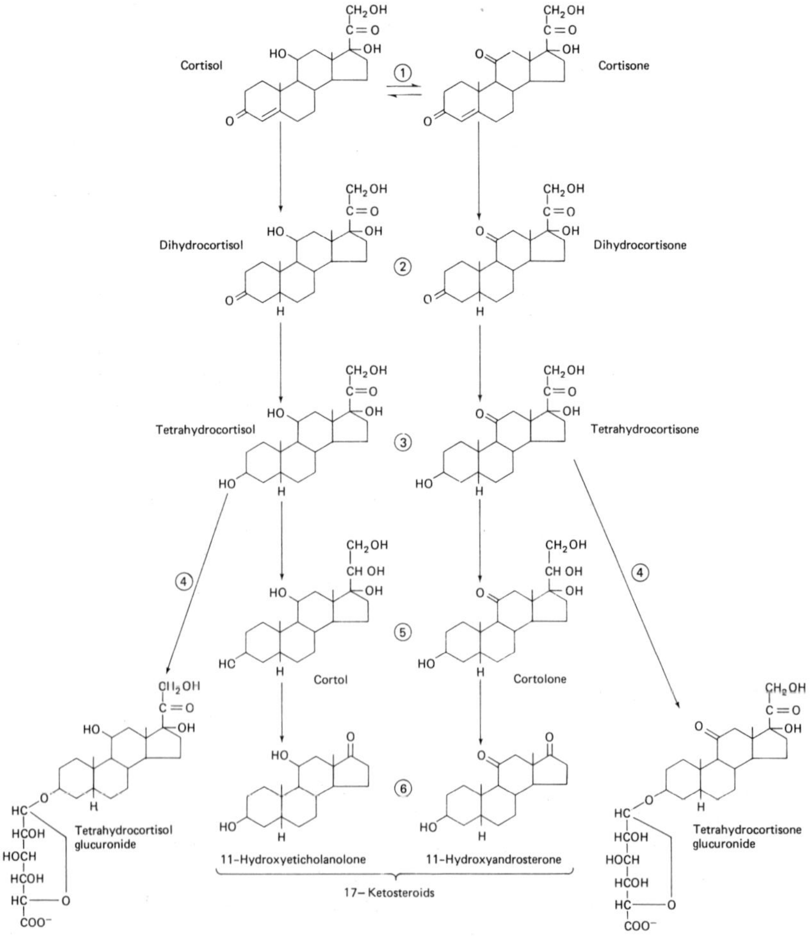

Fig. 9.3 Metabolic degradation of cortisol (see text). **N.B.** glucocorticoid metabolites are generally ketogenic steroids.

The pathways by which cortisol is metabolized are illustrated in Fig. 9.3 and the steps are identified by number in the following description. Some is converted to cortisone in the liver and possibly, to a very limited extent, in other tissues (1). No cortisone is secreted by the adrenal cortex itself and this conversion therefore represents the only source of endogenous cortisone. Both cortisone and cortisol are reduced in the liver or elsewhere to dihydrocortisone and dihydrocortisol respectively, with loss of the double bond between C4 and C5 in the A ring (2). These steroids are then hydroxylated at C3 to form tetrahydrocortisone and tetrahydrocortisol which reaction occurs exclusively in the liver (3). Most of these two tetrahydro-derivations are converted to glucuronides by conjugation at the C3-hydroxyl group (4). Glucuronidation occurs mainly in the liver and to a limited extent in the kidney. These water-soluble end-products are biologically inactive and are excreted almost entirely in the urine, virtually none appearing in the faeces. Some tetrahydrocortisol and tetrahydrocortisone is converted to the 17-ketosteroid precursors, cortol and cortolone, by reduction of the side chain at C18(5). 17-ketosteroids produced by oxidation of these steroids (6) have a weak androgenic effect but are devoid of glucocorticoid activity and appear in the urine mainly in the form of sulphate conjugates. These 17-ketosteroids differ from the principal androgen secreted by the zona reticularis, dehydroepiandrosterone, and from ketosteroids derived from testosterone by the possession of an = O or – OH group at C11 and are referred to collectively as 11-oxy-17-ketosteroids. In the normal human male, 17-ketosteroids of adrenal origin account for approximately 70 per cent of the total found in the urine and amount to about 10 mg/day. The remaining 30 per cent is derived from metabolism of testicular androgens. For reasons which are still obscure, the rate at which the liver inactivates glucocorticoids is depressed by several types of stress, which has the effect of increasing the concentration of these hormones in the plasma to higher levels than would occur in response to ACTH stimulation alone.

Mineralocorticoids

The MCR of aldosterone is approximately equal to total hepatic blood flow, indicating that this steroid, which is comparatively weakly bound to plasma protein, is completely cleared from the plasma as it passes through the liver. Here it is mainly converted to tetrahydroaldosterone glucuronide which is eliminated in the urine.

Actions on target tissues

Glucocorticoids

The glucocorticoids exert a multiplicity of actions on a wide range of tissues, the mechanisms of which are still poorly understood in many cases. They have an important role in the control of carbohydrate, fat, protein and purine metabolism and influence the function of the cardiovascular system, skeletal muscle, the central nervous system, lymphoid, connective and other tissues. They exert an important 'permissive' action and thereby influence the responses of many tissues to other hormones. They have a powerful anti-inflammatory effect and also increase the capacity to withstand almost any stress, whether it derives from the internal or external environment. In addition, during the last few years it has become clear that glucocorticoids released from the fetal adrenal, have a crucial role in the initiation of parturition, at least in certain species. These actions will now be discussed in detail.

Carbohydrate metabolism

The primary role of the glucocorticoids in the control of carbohydrate metabolism is to maintain the reserves of glycogen in the liver and, to a lesser extent, in the heart and skeletal muscle. Thus, administration of cortisol to normal animals has little or no immediate hyperglycaemic effect, although steroid diabetes can be produced in certain species, such as the rat, by repeated administration of large doses for prolonged periods. On the other hand, hypoglycaemia, due to adrenal insufficiency, is reversed by cortisol as liver glycogen is replenished. In adult animals, adrenalectomy does not normally lead to hypoglycaemia, provided that plenty of food is available to maintain the concentration of glycogen in the liver, but the animals are much more susceptible to starvation and become increasingly sensitive to insulin.

In contrast, removal of the adrenal glands from newborn animals results in fatal hypoglycaemia within a few hours in the absence of adequate replacement therapy. This is probably due to the fact that the peripheral tissues are particularly sensitive to insulin at this age as the rate at which insulin is released in these animals is considerably less than that in the adult.

A particularly striking example of the role of the glucocorticoids in the deposition of liver glycogen is provided by the late-term fetus. Jost and his colleagues in Paris have shown that during this stage of development, massive amounts of glycogen are laid down in the liver, due to the action of fetal adrenal steroids together with pituitary or placental growth hormone and prolactin. This reserve of carbohydrate is mobilized very rapidly during the first few hours after birth and serves as an energy source during the period in which the newborn animal is establishing a gastrointestinal route of absorption.

Glucocorticoids stimulate glycogen production by two separate gluconeogenic effects. First, they stimulate the breakdown of protein in skeletal muscle and the release of amino acids therefrom. Secondly, and paradoxically, they induce the formation of specific proteins in the liver. These proteins include enzymes such as the transaminases which catalyse the transfer of α-amino moieties to α-ketoglutarate, thereby providing a pathway for conversion to carbohydrate. This reaction also yields glutamic acid which leads to urea and purine biosynthesis. Thus there is a simultaneous increase in the release of amino acids from skeletal muscle and the rate at which these are 'trapped' by the liver and converted to carbohydrate. At the same time there is an increase in the activities of a number of other hepatic enzymes, such as fructose 1.6.diphosphatase and glucose.6.phosphatase, which tend to favour glucose production at the expense of glycolysis.

The glucocorticoids also exert an anti-insulin effect in peripheral tissues, effectively inhibiting glucose uptake, which explains why pancreatic diabetes is exacerbated by administration of these steroids and ameliorated by adrenalectomy. In adipose and lymphoid tissue the glucocorticoids directly oppose the action of insulin and thereby reduce glucose uptake. However, in skeletal muscle, the effect appears to be indirect, and is due to the rise in free fatty acids which occurs as a result of increased lipolysis *(see below)*, as the availability of excess free fatty acid limits the uptake and utilization of glucose in this tissue.

Protein metabolism
Normal growth depends upon the presence of glucocorticoids, possibly due to the loss of appetite and reduction in intestinal absorption which occurs in their absence. But excess of glucocorticoids causes a negative nitrogen balance due to catabolism of protein in the peripheral tissues. The effect is probably exacerbated by inhibition of protein anabolism and increased trapping of amino acids in the liver.

Fat metabolism
Glucocorticoids inhibit glucose uptake by adipose tissue, thereby reducing the availability of glycerophosphate for re-esterification of fatty acids and inhibiting lipogenesis. At the same time they appear to increase release of FFA directly. This effect depends upon synthesis of a protein, has a long latency and is blocked by actinomycin and puromycin. Glucocorticoids also control fat metabolism indirectly by potentiating the lipolytic response to other agents such as growth hormone or catecholamines. In the absence of glucocorticoids the lipolytic effects of these hormones are reduced to negligible proportions.

This provides one example of the numerous 'permissive' actions of the glucocorticoids. In each case the sensitivity of the tissue is greatly reduced in the absence of these steroids, which must therefore condition or sensitize the effector cells in some way. The hyperglycaemic response to adrenaline provides an example which can be understood more easily, since the steroids 'permit' release of glucose from the liver by replenishing the available glycogen.

Circulatory system
Corticosteroids are essential for maintenance of normal circulatory function and adrenalectomy leads to circulatory collapse. This is due mainly to impaired myocardial function, together with a fall in peripheral vascular resistance. The primary cardiac defect appears to reside in the contractile proteins as there is a pronounced loss of ATPase activity, which is corrected by administration of dexamethasone. Concentrations of Na^+ and K^+ are maintained even though renal transport mechanisms may be defective. In the periphery, the mineralocorticoids, but not the glucocorticoids, exert a 'permissive' effect on the vasoconstrictor effects of catecholamines. This is associated with the maintenance of normal internal Na^+ concentration in the smooth muscle of the tunica media and may explain the reduction in peripheral resistance.

Skeletal muscle
Glucorticoids are indispensible to the maintenance of muscular activity, and even to life itself during severe exercise, but the mechanisms involved are still

obscure. Neither the maintenance of normal glucose nor electrolyte concentrations in the plasma and extracellular fluid can compensate for the absence of these steroids. Insufficiency causes rapid muscular fatigue and excess leads to muscular atrophy, due to protein catabolism. No doubt these steroids are implicated in a multitude of biochemical reactions, both directly and 'permissively', but a major factor which affects the work capacity of skeletal muscle deprived of glucocorticoids in intact animals is undoubtedly circulatory failure.

A further possibility is that adrenocortical insufficiency leads to increased fragility of the lysosomes in skeletal muscle (see under 'Anti-inflammatory effects'). Release of acid hydrolases from these subcellular particles during muscular activity might help to explain some of the deleterious effects of exercise under these conditions.

Nervous system

The brain is extremely sensitive to glucocorticoids and variations within the normal physiological range produce detectable changes in the threshold to certain sensations as well as higher functions, such as concentration, memory and intellectual performance. The phenomenon of 'jet-lag' may be due to precisely these changes, which occur as a consequence of disturbing the normal circadian rhythm in such a way that maximum rates of cortisol secretion occur at an unaccustomed time of day.

In general, glucocorticoid deficiency depresses cerebral activity, causing apathy and lassitude, while excess produces a state of euphoria, insomnia and hyperactivity. Overt psychosis may result from excess, but is almost invariably reversible.

Cerebral blood flow is reduced in adrenocortical insufficiency. This is probably a local manifestation of generalized circulatory failure and is reversed by administration of cortisol, but not mineralocorticoids. Vascular failure may well account for depression of cerebral function under these conditions and may also explain why adrenalectomized animals exhibit convulsions and fits more readily than normal animals in response to such stimuli as hypoglycaemia, hypoxia or acidosis. The mechanism whereby glucocorticoids increase the excitability of the brain is unknown. Administration of large doses of mineralocorticoids to animals decreases the excitability of the brain due to changes in electrolyte concentration.

> Henkin has shown that adrenalectomy or adrenocortical insufficiency causes a marked reduction in the threshold to such sensations as taste, smell and hearing—detection being increased by a factor of 100 for taste, 1000 for olfaction and by 13 dB in the case of hearing. Administration of glucocorticoids, but not mineralocorticoids, restores these thresholds to normal and each is depressed by excess of glucocorticoid. However, as these thresholds rise, in the absence of the adrenal steroids, the ability to recognize and distinguish between the signals diminishes. These changes are believed to depend on the effects of the glucocorticoids on nervous conduction, which are to reduce the rate at which the action potential is propagated along the nerve axon but to increase the speed of synaptic transmission. The consequences of glucocorticoid deprivation are, therefore, increased speed of axonal conduction with prolongation of synaptic transmission. These changes will affect the timing by which the sensory impulses

arrive at the sensory cortex, resulting in the observed failure of discrimination. The reduction in sensory threshold is tentatively attributed to some change in central nervous excitability to these particular sensory modalities.

Lymphoid and connective tissue

One of the most characteristic signs of adrenocortical insufficiency is hyperplasia of lymphoid tissue and increase in circulating lymphocytes. In the normal animal, the adrenal glucocorticoids provide a check to the growth of this tissue and are responsible for regression of the thymus during the neonatal period. Administration of cortisol causes rapid dissolution of lymphoid tissue, which is reflected by a lymphocytopenia which is often discernible within fifty to sixty minutes. Mitosis is inhibited, lymphocyte nuclei become pyknotic and the cells lose their cytoplasm, which is promptly phagocytosed.

> There is a greater relative conversion of protein to amino acids in lymphocytes than any other tissue under the influence of adrenal steroids, although the absolute contribution to total energy production is comparatively small.
>
> The glucocorticoids directly inhibit glucose uptake by lymphocytes, but it is thought that their principal action is depletion of nucleic acids and inhibition of DNA synthesis in these cells. It has been suggested that steroids influence lymphocyte maturation by the following mechanism. The cells contain a 11β-hydroxydehydrogenase which converts cortisol to cortisone in the presence of DPN and TPN in immature lymphocytes and, since cortisone is relatively inactive, protects them from dissolution. Predominance of reduced coenzymes (DPNH and TPNH) in mature lymphocytes leads to the reverse reaction, and conversion of cortisone to cortisol leads to cellular destruction.

Glucocorticoids exert pronounced effects on connective tissue, for which reason they are widely used clinically to inhibit fibrosis, and in the various collagen diseases. Cortisol inhibits the synthesis of mucopolysaccharides and increases the degree of polymerization of hyaluronic acid, thereby substantially modifying the composition of the ground substance. It also produces specific morphological changes in the fibroblasts, which may become epithelioid in appearance and resistant to the normal degenerative changes associated with inflammation.

Anti-inflammatory effect

The increase in vascular permeability which occurs in inflammation is due mainly to histamine release and has been shown to be independent of any venous congestion. Mast cells represent the principal source of histamine in the tissues and the numbers of these at any site of injury are substantially reduced by glucocorticoids, as is the release of histamine from these cells. In addition, the cellular response in inflammation is modified by the glucocorticoids as follows.

1. The number of circulating polymorphonuclear leucocytes increases, but their stickiness, phagocytic and digestive activity are reduced.
2. Lymphocytopenia (see above).
3. Phagocytotic and digestive activity of the monocytes is reduced.
4. The rate of division and multiplication of the plasma cells is reduced, thereby reducing antibody formation in response to primary antigenic stimuli.

Glucocorticoids may also exert an important anti-inflammatory effect by stabilizing lysosome membranes, as first suggested by Weissman and Thomas who showed that the toxic effects of excessive doses of vitamin A, which 'labilizes' lysosomal membranes, are prevented by pretreatment with cortisol. Lysosomes contain powerful acid hydrolases and appear to represent an intracellular digestive system which is particularly well developed in phagocytic cells. The specific granules of polymorphonuclear leucocytes are lysosomes, the acid hydrolases of which are discharged into the phagocytic vacuoles to initiate the digestive process when particles are engulfed. Cellular damage and rupture of lysosomes leads to the release of substances which produce inflammation, causing increased vasodilation and vascular permeability, and this process could be substantially reduced by the stabilizing effect of the glucocorticoids.

The glucocorticoids also inhibit the formation of various kinins, such as bradykinin, from the appropriate α-globulin by inhibiting the enzyme kallikrein. This action may also be important in the control of the inflammatory response by limiting the production of irritant peptides.

The number of circulating eosinophils, like the lymphocytes, is strikingly reduced by administration of either ACTH or cortisol. This is due to increased uptake of these cells by the spleen and lungs and has frequently been used as an index of ACTH release. Unfortunately, it can be misleading, as variations in the eosinophil count are now known to occur in response to various stresses in adrenalectomized animals.

ACTH secretion
The glucorticoids strongly inhibit the release of ACTH from the anterior pituitary. This effect represents an important negative feedback and is discussed in detail under 'Control of secretion'.

Water metabolism
A deficiency of the adrenal glucocorticoids leads to an inability to dispose of a water load and consequent susceptibility to water intoxication. This appears to be due mainly to a reduction in glomerular filtration rate (GFR), although an increase in the concentration of antidiuretic hormone in the plasma has also been described. Administration of cortisol, but not aldosterone, restores water diuresis by increasing GFR.

Parturition
In sheep a rapid increase in the rate of cortisol secretion by the fetal adrenal gland occurs at the end of gestation and serves to initiate parturition. Cortisol acts on the placenta by stimulating the conversion of progesterone to oestrogen. The consequential decline in plasma progesterone and increase in oestrogen secretion induces a rise in the concentration of PGF 2α (see p.145) in the maternal cotyledons and myometrium. This prostaglandin sensitizes the myometrium to the action of oxytocin (see p.60) and may also have some direct oxytoxic effect. A similar sequence of events is believed to occur in other species, such as the cow and goat, but it has not yet been established whether parturition is initiated in the same way in the human.

For convenience, the peripheral actions of glucocorticoids are summarized in Table 9.2.

Table 9.2   Summary of the peripheral actions of the adrenal glucocorticoids

Tissue	Action	Mechanism
Liver	Maintenance of glycogen reserve by gluconeogenesis	Increased trapping of amino acids and conversion to α-ketogluterate by tyrosine transaminase ↑ fructose -1.6. diphosphatase and glucose-6-phosphatase
Skeletal muscle	i. Loss of structural protein and atrophy	↑ Protein catabolism; ↓ Protein anabolism
	ii. Insufficiency leads to rapid fatigue	Maintenance of cardio-vascular function
Fat	Lipolysis	↓ Glucose uptake; ↑ FFA release; potentiate glycolytic actions of catecholamines and growth hormone
Heart	Maintenance of force of contraction	Unknown
Peripheral vasculature	Necessary for normal vasoconstrictor responses	Potentiate vasoconstrictor effects of catecholamines
Nervous system	Required for maintenance of normal cerebral activity	Deficiency causes depression and excess causes hyperactivity
Sensation	Affect both threshold of detection and discriminatory capacity	Decrease speed of axonal conduction and increase rate of synaptic transmission
Lymphoid tissue	Dissolution and regression	i. ↓ Glucose uptake; ii. deplete nucleic acid and inhibit DNA synthesis
Connective tissue	Inhibition	i. Inhibit synthesis of ground substance; ii. inhibit growth and development of fibroblasts

Table 9.2 (cont.)

Tissue	Action	Mechanism
Inflammation	Inhibition	i. decreased activity and production of various leucocytes; ii. inhibit kinin formation; iii. stablilize lysosomol membranes
Pituitary/ hypothalamus	Inhibit ACTH secretion	i. Direct effect on pituitary corticotrophs; ii. inhibition of CRF release from the hypothalamus
Kidney	Maintain capacity to excrete water	Maintain a normal glomeruler filtration rate
Placenta	Initiation of parturition in certain species	↓ Placentral progesterone production ; ↑ placental oestrogen production

Mineralocorticoids

Aldosterone is the principal mineralocorticoid which is secreted by the adrenal and is also by far the most potent. It promotes reabsorption of Na^+ from urine, sweat, saliva and gastrointestinal contents and probably promotes Na^+/K^+ exchange across cell membranes, to some extent in all tissues. Its most important physiological action is that which it exerts on the renal tubules, since electrolyte excretion is normally controlled by this means. Aldosterone acts on the distal convoluted tubule to promote reabsorption of Na^+ in exchange for K^+ or H^+. There is also some quite recent evidence suggesting that aldosterone may also promote reabsorption of Na^+ in the proximal convoluted tubule; the effect of aldosterone on active transport of Na^+ is so widespread that the cells of the proximal convoluted tubule would be unique if they were found to be completely unresponsive to the hormone. Stimulation of K^+ excretion by aldosterone is largely dependent upon sodium status and the excretion of K^+ in response to aldosterone is virtually abolished in animals deprived of sodium.

Prolonged administration of aldosterone leads to potassium depletion and replacement of part of the potassium lost from the intracellular fluid compartment by sodium. The concentration of Na^+ in the plasma is not altered greatly because water is retained with sodium and serves to expand the volume of the extracellular fluid. However, oedema is comparatively rare because the kidney usually 'escapes' from the sodium-retaining influence of the hormone, although potassium excretion is maintained. 'Escape' from the sodium-retaining effect of aldosterone, under these conditions, is thought to be due to the rise in glomerular filtration rate which results from expansion of extracellular fluid volume.

There is also evidence that administration of aldosterone leads to increased excretion of both Ca^{2+} and Mg^{2+} in the urine, but it seems that both effects are secondary responses to expansion of extracellular fluid. In dogs treated with exogenous deoxycorticosterone, sodium retention increases within twenty-four hours, whereas increased excretion of the divalent cations is not observed for several days.

The precise mechanism whereby mineralocorticoids stimulate the active transport of Na^+ is still not completely understood, but most of the evidence suggests that it involves activation of DNA to produce a form of RNA which regulates the synthesis of some specific protein. This protein may be an enzyme which regulates the rate of oxidative phosphorylation whereby energy for active transport is provided. Alternatively, it may act by facilitating entry of Na^+ into the cell, which in turn stimulates cellular metabolism linked to the sodium pump. However, it is generally accepted that these hormones act by inducing protein synthesis, as do the glucocorticoids, which explains the long delay between stimulus and response. In contrast, the effect of aldosterone on K^+ excretion is thought to be independent of protein synthesis and persists after treatment with actinomycin D.

Effects of deficiency

Absolute adrenal cortical deficiency can be produced experimentally, either surgically or pharmacologically.

Drugs such as metyrapone or amphenone B block the synthesis of both glucocorticoids and mineralocorticoids by inhibiting hydroxylation. A more specific deficiency is produced by administration of mitotane (o,p'-DDD), which has a relatively selective cytotoxic action on the cells of the zona fasciculata and thus reduces secretion of glucocorticoids, or spironolactone, which has a similar structure to aldosterone and inhibits the action of that hormone by competing with it for the available receptor sites.

Adrenal cortical deficiency in man occurs in **Addison's disease**. It is a comparatively rare condition which may arise as a result of tubercular or neoplastic damage to the adrenal gland or auto-immune disease. Complete loss of adrenal cortical function would rapidly cause death, but the defect develops insidiously over a prolonged period and patients generally have a relative rather than an absolute deficiency (Daggett: *Clinical Endocrinology,* Chapter 5). Adrenal insufficiency can also arise as a result of defective release of ACTH from the pituitary, in which case the symptoms are entirely attributable to lack of glucocorticoids and control of salt and water metabolism is well maintained.

The symptoms of Addison's disease are entirely attributable to lack of adrenal corticoids, and therefore explicable in terms of the various actions of these steroids described above. The chronic disease is characterized by weakness, loss of weight and appetite, hypotension and a reduction in heart size. The patients are easily fatigued, apathetic and may exhibit spontaneous hypoglycaemia. Increased pigmentation of the skin is one of the most characteristic features of the disease and appears to be due to the melanocyte-stimulating activity of ACTH, which is secreted in excessive amounts from the anterior pituitary.

The pituitary-adrenal axis is exquisitely sensitive to a wide variety of 'stresses'; a rapid increase in cortisol secretion is one of the earliest detectable responses to such stimuli and generally precedes release of adrenaline from the adrenal medulla. It is still not clear precisely how the glucocorticoids ameliorate the effects of stress, although their importance in this regard is undeniable and is reflected in the fact that moderate stress often causes complete collapse due to an acute adrenal crisis in chronic Addisonian patients.

Acute adrenal crisis is a state of general collapse. There may be almost any combination of gastrointestinal symptoms, such as nausea, vomiting and diarrhoea, or hypoglycaemia, dehydration, haemoconcentration and hypotension and, without adequate treatment, death will usually occur from circulatory collapse.

Effects of excess

Glucocorticoid excess in man produces quite characteristic clinical symptoms, which were first described by Harvey Cushing in 1932: these symptoms can be largely explained in terms of the actions of the glucocorticoids discussed above. **Cushing's syndrome** may arise as a result of adrenal tumours, excess secretion of ACTH from any cause, or administration of large doses of exogenous glucocorticoids for prolonged periods (Daggett: *Clinical Endocrinology*, Chapter 5). Resorption of fat in the extremities, combined with deposition of fat in the face and trunk, produces the so-called 'moon-faced' appearance and 'buffalo hump'. These are usually associated with the appearance of purple striae over the abdomen, thighs and upper arms as the subcutaneous tissues are stretched and even ruptured. Wounds heal poorly, with inadequate fibrous tissue replacement, and hair growth is inhibited. Glucocorticoids inhibit the action of vitamin D, increase excretion of calcium in the urine by raising glomerular filtration rate, and cause increased catabolism of protein; these actions together lead to dissolution of bone. Protein depletion causes wasting of skeletal muscle and thinning of the skin. Increased gluconeogenesis associated with reduced peripheral utilization of glucose predisposes to diabetes, which frequently becomes overt in individuals who are genetically disposed to that disease (see Chapter 4). The amounts of glucocorticoid secreted are usually sufficiently large to cause salt and water retention and potassium depletion, but oedema is not a prominent feature of the disease, due to the increase in glomerular filtration rate. Hypertension, however, is common.

Excess production of aldosterone was first described by Conn in 1955. His patient was a 35-year-old woman with an adrenal cortical tumour who made a complete recovery when the tumour was removed. Typically, the symptoms of primary aldosteronism, or **Conn's syndrome**, are all attributable to mineralocorticoid excess (Daggett: *Clinical Endocrinology*, Chapter 5). These include sodium and water retention, potassium loss, metabolic alkalosis, polyuria, polydipsia and hypertension. The ratio of Na:K in sweat, saline and urine is depressed, while the intracellular concentration of sodium rises at the expense of potassium as all the sodium/potassium exchange mechanisms which are affected by aldosterone are maximally stimulated. In the renal tubules, Na$^+$ is reabsorbed in exchange for either K$^+$ or H$^+$, causing an initial loss of K$^+$ from the extracellular fluid. The extracellular K$^+$ concentration is effectively maintained, however, by diffusion from the comparatively enormous intracellular reservoir of K$^+$ and the change in plasma K$^+$ concentration is comparatively small. Continued depletion of this reserve eventually leads to increased diffusion of Na$^+$ and H$^+$ into the cells and a progressive increase in renal excretion of H$^+$ in exchange for Na$^+$. Prolonged exposure to excess aldosterone therefore produces a hypokalaemic alkalosis with excretion of an acid urine.

It should be noted that the increased amount of Na$^+$ in the plasma and extracellular fluid (ECF) osmotically withdraws an equivalent volume of water from the intracellular compartment and the glomerular filtrate as it passes through the renal tubules. This has the effect of expanding the volume of the extracellular fluid without significantly increasing the concentration of Na$^+$ therein. A more puzzling feature of Conn's syndrome is the fact that oedema occurs comparatively rarely. This may be due in part to the phenomenon of aldosterone escape, referred to previously (see p.128) and accounted for by the fact that expansion of the extracellular fluid volume eventually leads to such an increase in glomerular filtration rate that urinary excretion of Na$^+$ is restored to normal, in spite of the high rate of reabsorption in the tubules. Such a mechanism might restrict the change in volume of the ECF and thereby prevent overt oedema. Entry of Na$^+$ into cells depleted of K$^+$ would act in the same direction. Finally, a natriuretic hormone has been postulated which might be released in response to Na$^+$ retention.

Hyperaldosteronism also occurs in association with liver disease, where it is thought to be caused by defective metabolism of the hormone, and in disorders in which there is a reduction in effective blood volume leading to inappropriate stimulation of aldosterone release.

Androgens and oestrogens

Excess adrenal androgens may be secreted either as a result of some congenital metabolic disturbance or an adrenal tumour, the latter being very rare. A variety of clinical symptoms may be produced, depending on which steroid is dominant. Thus, feminization may occur as a result of excess oestrogens secreted by adrenal tumours, although it is extremely rare. More commonly, such tumours produce an excess of androgens which will cause precocious puberty in children and masculinization in the female, but no obvious symptoms in the adult male (Daggett: *Clinical Endocrinology*, Chapter 5).

Control of secretion

Glucocorticoids

The control of glucocorticoid secretion will be discussed in relation to the components of the hypothalamo-pituitary-adrenocortical axis as illustrated and numbered in Fig. 9.4.

1. *The action of ACTH on the adrenal cortex*
Adrenocorticotrophin (corticotrophin, see p.78) is the only known stimulus to

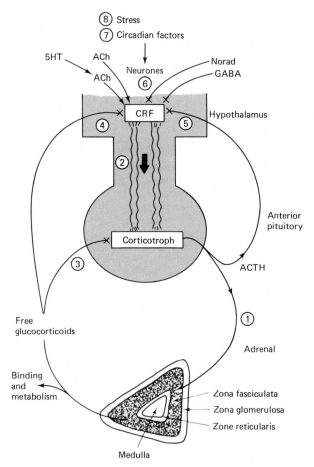

Fig. 9.4 The hypothalamo – pituitary – adrenocortical axis (see text). ACh = acetylcholine; norad = noradrenaline; 5HT = 5-hydroxytryptamine; **GABA**, γ-amino-butyric acid; → = stimulation; ⇥ = inhibition.

glucocorticoid secretion under physiological conditions: its effects on steroidogenesis are discussed on p.117. Intravenous administration of ACTH in a dose as low as 0.5 ng/kg body weight produces an increase in glucocorticoid release within two to three minutes. Increasing the dose of ACTH elevates steroid output to a maximum, after which further increase in ACTH serves only to prolong the effect.

2. *Stimulation of ACTH secretion*
Attempts to isolate the hypophysiotrophic hormone which stimulates ACTH secretion (CRF) have been unsuccessful (p.73). It now seems unlikely that vasopressin is normally implicated.

3. and **4.** *Glucocorticoid feedback*
Glucocorticoids suppress ACTH secretion; thus ACTH concentration in blood increases after adrenalectomy and in Addison's disease and is decreased in response to exogenous steroids. This feedback can be shown, by local administration, to occur both at the pituitary and at the hypothalamic level.

There appear to be two components to the feedback at each level; a fast feedback (FFB) and a delayed feedback (DFB). Fast feedback occurs immediately and is related to the rate of change of steroid concentration: it appears to be the result of inhibition of *release* of ACTH and/or CRF: the inhibition is short lived. Delayed feedback is delayed in onset, not reaching its maximum inhibitory effect until one to two hours after steroid administration: the degree of inhibition is related to the stable level of steroid attained. Delayed feedback seems to be due to impairment in the *synthesis* of ACTH and/or CRF. Such a combination of rate-sensitive (FFB) and proportional (DFB) control conveys increased sophistication to our conception of feedback regulation of adrenal cortical activity and may well prove to be present elsewhere in the endocrine system.

5. *Action of ACTH on CRF secretion*
Short-loop feedback does not seem to be present in the thyroid axis (p.107), but there is some evidence to suggest that ACTH in the concentrations achieved during stress (see below) may modulate CRF secretion.

6. *Neural control of CRF*
More is probably known of the neural factors involved in CRF release than for other releasing hormones. Neuropharmacological evidence indicates that the CRF-releasing neurones are excited directly by ACh-releasing neurones and indirectly by neurones releasing 5HT (see Fig. 9.4). Inhibitory neurones are of two types (noradrenaline or γ-amino-butyric acid (GABA) releasing). Such information could have considerable clinical implication and may lead to new methods of treating Cushing's syndrome due to ACTH-secreting pituitary tumours.

7. *Circadian factors*
Glucocorticoid output shows a diurnal fluctuation, this is of neural origin and thus involves a parallel fluctuation in ACTH and CRF release. The source of the rhythm appears to be in the suprachiasmic nucleus of the hypothalamus and is entrained to the dark/light cycle.

8. *Stress*
Stress is a term which, in the physiological sense, embraces a variety of circumstances in which an animal's internal or external environment becomes disturbed to an extent where normal homeostatic or behavioural responses are insufficient to correct the disturbance. Examples of potential or actual stresses include hypoglycaemia, hypoxia, asphyxia, hypotension, haemorrhage, extremes of environmental temperature or pressure, injury, infection, anaesthesia and surgery. Another category of stress is psychological stress, of which modern man is subject to an almost limitless variety! All stresses

promote ACTH secretion, although some may also stimulate the release of other hormones such as adrenaline and growth hormone.

The purpose of stress-induced ACTH release remains somewhat of an enigma. While it is clear that animals in which the adrenocortical axis is defective are peculiarly susceptible to stress, it remains to be resolved *how* glucocorticoids help protect the animal against such a wide variety of stressful factors.

Mineralocorticoids

The rate of synthesis and release of aldosterone from the zona glomerulosa can be influenced by a number of factors, most important of which are the peptide, angiotensin II (see below), ACTH, high plasma $[K^+]$ and low plasma $[Na^+]$. All these factors are believed to act by increasing production of cholesterol to pregnenolone (see Fig. 9.2). In addition, long-term salt deprivation also stimulates aldosterone secretion by promoting conversion of corticosterone to aldosterone: this effect does not involve cAMP. Of the factors which can be shown experimentally to influence aldosterone secretion, angiotensin II is currently held to be the most important and will therefore be discussed in detail below. However, the other factors merit brief mention.

ACTH

The importance of this hormone is species dependent. In the rat the anterior pituitary is essential to the aldosterone response to sodium depletion, but in man ACTH appears much less important. It is probably fair to say that in man ACTH exerts a 'permissive' effect on the zona glomerulosa by ensuring the maintenance of adequate steroid precursors for aldosterone, but it probably plays little part in the short-term control of aldosterone, except when released in large amounts in response to severe stress. It should be noted, however, that ACTH can influence aldosterone output indirectly by promoting the release of cortisol and corticosterone which, although only possessing less than 1/500th of the mineralocorticoid effect of aldosterone, can exert significant salt-retaining effects when present in large quantities (see p.130).

Potassium ions

Increase in plasma $[K^+]$ (hyperkalaemia) can produce a rapid increase in aldosterone secretion rate, e.g. increase in $[K^+]$ from $4-5$ mEq/l to $7-8$ mEq/l can cause up to a tenfold increase in aldosterone concentration within fifteen to forty-five minutes. Some of this effect may be via the renin-angiotensin system (Fig. 9.5) but, since it persists even after nephrectomy and can be shown *in vitro* in perfused adrenals, it must in part be due to a direct effect on the glomerulosa cells. In normal circumstances it is unlikely that the plasma $[K^+]$ changes sufficiently to produce significant changes in aldosterone secretion.

Sodium ions

Acute decrease in plasma $[Na^+]$ (hyponatraemia) will cause increased aldosterone secretion. However, this particular stimulus has powerful effects

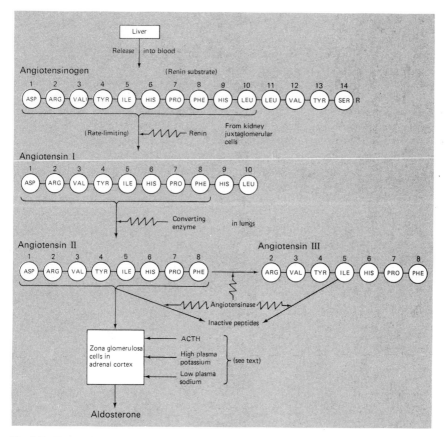

Fig. 9.5 The renin-angiotensin system.

via the renin-angiotensin system which would certainly over-ride any direct effect on the glomerulosa cells. Nevertheless, such a direct effect is probably present since hyponatraemia is an effective stimulus even after nephrectomy and under *in vitro* conditions.

The renin-angiotensin system
Figure 9.8 illustrates the essential elements of the so-called renin-angiotensin system for control of aldosterone secretion.

The liver releases into the blood an α_2-globulin containing 14 amino acids, called angiotensinogen or renin substrate peptide. Renin (a proteolytic enzyme of mol.wt. 42 000) is secreted by the juxtaglomerular cells in the kidney and cleaves the angiotensinogen molecule leaving the decapeptide angiotensin I. This in turn loses two further amino acids due to the action of converting enzyme, which occurs mainly in the lungs. The resulting octapeptide, angiotensin II, is responsible for stimulating the increased synthesis and release of aldosterone from the cells of the zona glomerulosa. Angiotensin II has a very short half-life for it is rapidly inactivated by peptidases in plasma, but one breakdown product, the heptapeptide angiotensin III, has residual physiological activity.

Normally, the rate-limiting step in the series of events described above and illustrated in Fig. 9.5 is the production of angiotensin I by the action of renin. As a first approximation, therefore, the rate of aldosterone secretion is effectively determined by the rate of secretion of renin from the juxtaglomerular cells (the availability of angiotensinogen could also be limiting to the process and much work is now being done on the control of its production, but little is yet known about it). The juxtaglomerular cells are modified smooth muscle cells in the tunica media of the afferent anteriole (Fig. 9.6). They contain membrane-bound granules of renin and are closely opposed to the **macula densa**, which is a region of modified tubule cells found at the point where the distal convoluted tubule bends back to approach its own glomerulus (Fig. 9.6). The juxtaglomerular apparatus includes both juxtaglomerular cells and macula densa. Sympathetic nerve fibres end close to or on the juxtaglomerular cells and also have a vasoconstrictor effect on the afferent arteriole.

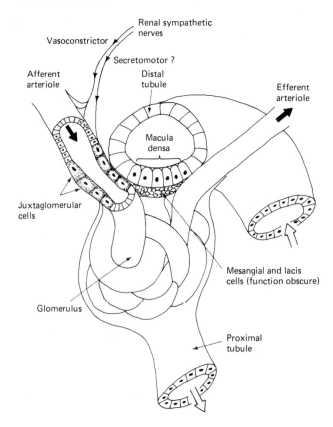

Fig. 9.6 Schematic representation of the juxtaglomerular apparatus and associated structures.

What then dictates the rate of release of renin from the juxtaglomerular cells? This is a question which has generated and still generates a controversy in which more heat than light has been produced. What is generally agreed is that renin release is stimulated under the following circumstances.

1. Decrease in renal perfusion pressure (e.g. following a decrease in systemic arterial pressure or narrowing of the renal artery).
2. Decrease in ECF volume (e.g. after haemorrhage).
3. Apparent decrease in ECF volume (constriction of the inferior vena cava).
4. Sodium depletion (low sodium intake or use of diuretics causing sodium loss).
5. β-adrenergic agents.

It is clear that, under physiological conditions, *none* of the above factors would, in isolation, control renin release. Nevertheless, alone or in combination, the circumstances enumerated above would find appropriate homeostatic compensation in the activation of the renin-angiotensin axis. Thus, sodium conservation and the consequent increase in ECF volume, together with possible pressor effects of angiotensin, constitute a powerful weapon in situations of cardiovascular emergency.

Androgens and oestrogens

The quantities of sex steroids secreted by the zona reticularis are normally negligible and little is known of factors other than ACTH which promote steroidogenesis.

Further reading

Daggett, Peter (1981). *Clinical Endocrinology*. Edward Arnold, London.
Davis, J. O. and Freeman, R. H. (1976). Mechanisms regulating renin release. *Physiology Review* **56**, 1.
Gower, D. B. (1979). *Steroid hormones*. Croom Helm, London.
Greep, R. O. and Astwood, E. B. (1975). Endocrinology: Handbook of Physiology Vol. VI. *Adrenal Gland*. American Physiological Society, Washington.
James, V. H. T., Serio, M., Giusti, G. and Martini, L. (Eds.) (1978). *The endocrine function of the human adrenal cortex*. Academic Press, London.
Nelson, D. H. (1980). *The Adrenal Cortex*. W. B. Saunders, London.
Reid, I. A., Morris, B. J. and Ganong, W. F. (1978). The renin-angiotensin system. *Annual Review of Physiology* **40**, 377.

10

Other endocrine actions

The pineal gland

The pineal gland releases the indole **melatonin**. The rate of release is variable and in some mammals is related to environmental lighting. Many functions have been attributed to melatonin but, of these, only effects on sexual maturation and ovarian function can at present be substantiated.

Anatomy and microstructure

The pineal, or epiphysis cerebri, is an outgrowth from the roof of the third ventricle richly innervated by sympathetic nerve fibres and by some parasympathetic fibres. In submammalian vertebrates it may contain sensory cells (e.g. the 'third eye' of certain reptiles), but the mammalian pineal is devoid of sensory cells. For many years, therefore, the mammalian pineal was considered a 'vestigial' organ, but there is now general acceptance that it does have an endocrine role, although there remains considerable disagreement about the significance of this function.

The secretory cells of the pineal (pinealocytes) possess elongated processes which terminate in knob-like structures on the blood vessels, suggesting the pathway for the release of melatonin into the circulation (it is also possible that melatonin may be released directly into the CSF).

The pineal is particularly prominent in young animals, but normally begins to shrink around the time of puberty, after which deposits of calcium and magnesium phosphate appear in the gland. This 'pineal sand' often enables the gland to be clearly delineated in radiographs. In adult man the gland weighs about 120 mg.

Chemistry and metabolism of hormone

The principal pineal hormone is the indole N-acetyl-5-methoxytryptamine (melatonin; Fig. 10.1). This substance, unlike its precursor serotonin, seems to be synthesized exclusively by the pineal. Thus its concentration in the gland and that of the enzyme catalysing the final stage of its synthesis, hydroxyindole-O-methyltransferase (HIOMT), provide a valuable index of

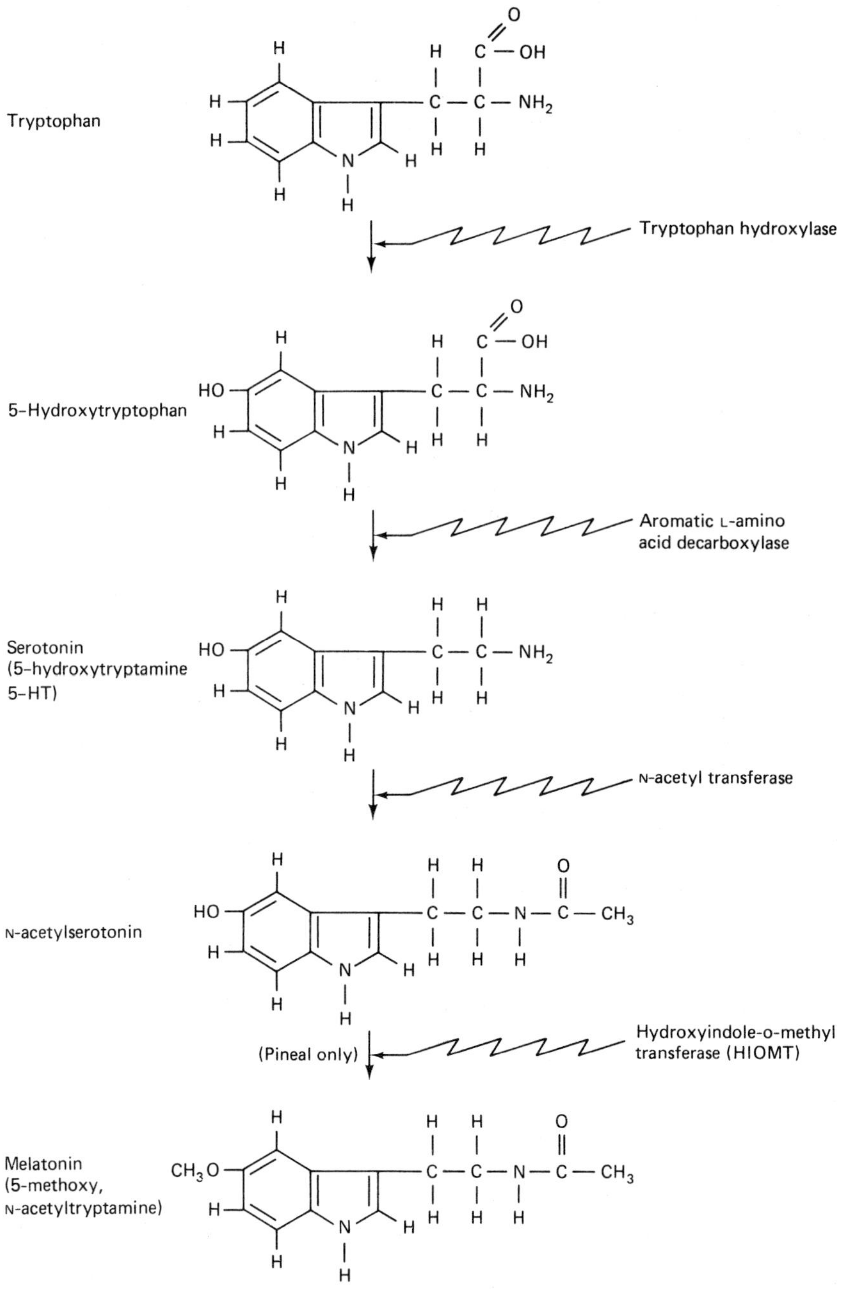

Fig. 10.1 The biosynthesis of melatonin in the pineal gland.

pineal function. Other related indoles present may prove to be physiologically important and some authorities also claim that polypeptide pineal hormones are of significance.

Effect on target tissues

The principal action of melatonin appears to be on the reproductive hormones (antigonadotrophic actions). In rats and hamsters, melatonin administration inhibits ovulation and the associated increase in plasma luteinizing hormone concentration. This action appears to be at the level of the hypothalamus by an inhibition of the neural mechanisms controlling LHRF secretion. Chronic administration of melatonin also delays puberty in rats. The pineal gland plays a part in the control of seasonal reproductive rhythms of certain subprimate species by virtue of the effect of environmental lighting (see below). Although it remains unclear whether there are specific pineal antigonadotrophic hormones, pineal activity appears to augment the secretion of prolactin by suppressing hypothalamic secretion of prolactin-inhibitory factor (PIF).

Other effects claimed for pineal hormones include suppression of the secretion of growth hormone, TSH and ACTH.

Effect of deficiency

Total pinealectomy in experimental animals produces variable results, due to species differences and nonspecific side effects incidental to the operation. However, puberty tends to occur earlier in such animals and reproductive rhythms dependent upon environmental light (see p.141) are disturbed. Precocious puberty is also seen in humans with certain pineal tumours (non-parenchymatous) where melotonin secretion is probably depressed. One can tentatively speculate that hypofunction of the pineal, by decreasing the anti-gonadotrophic actions of melatonin, permits puberty to occur earlier.

Effect of excess

Pineal hyperfunction in man (pinealoma) and melatonin treatment in weanling rats causes a delay in puberty or secondary regression of gonadal activity in postpubertal individuals, thus supporting the general hypothesis that the pineal exerts an antigonadotrophic effect.

Control of secretion

The formation of melatonin fluctuates in experimental animals in relation to environmental lighting. Thus light tends to suppress melatonin formation while darkness enhances it.

The pathway is complex but, in essence, is as follows (Fig. 10.2). Light stimulates the retinal receptors, impulses pass initially along the inferior accessory optic tract to the brain and spinal cord centres influencing sympathetic nervous activity, and thence to the pineal via sympathetic nerves

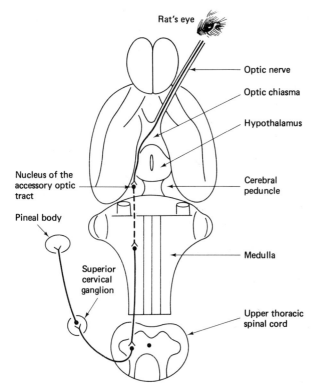

Rat's eye

Optic nerve

Optic chiasma

Hypothalamus

Nucleus of the
accessory optic
tract

Cerebral
peduncle

Pineal body

Medulla

Superior
cervical
ganglion

Upper thoracic
spinal cord

Fig. 10.2 Diagram to demonstrate the nerve pathways connecting the retina to the pineal of the rat. (With permission from Wurtman, R. J., Axelrod, J. and Kelly, D. E. (1968). *The Pineal*. Copyright by Academic Press, Inc. London.)

originating in the superior cervical ganglion: activity in these nerves suppresses melatonin synthesis. In darkness, this inhibitory pathway is inactive and melatonin synthesis takes place. Evidence to support this theory has been obtained from experiments in which animals were kept in continuous darkness or continuous light: the melatonin and HIOMT content of the pineals altered as predicted.

On the basis of this model for pineal control, it is currently held that the pineal plays a role in influencing reproductive patterns in seasonally breeding animals where sexual competence can be related to day length. It probably also exerts an influence by virtue of its diurnal changes in activity, in the regulation of shorter-term oestrus and menstrual cycles, although detailed evidence to support this idea is still lacking.

The thymus gland

The endocrine role of the thymus gland is unclear. Nevertheless, thymic hormones appear to be implicated in the sequence of events resulting in the development of the immunological reactivity of certain lymphoid cells, particularly the T (thymus-dependent) cells.

Anatomy and microstructure of gland

The thymus is situated in the anterior mediastinum in close association with the pericardium and great veins. It is relatively much larger in the fetus and child than in the adult, for it undergoes a marked involution at the time of puberty. The outer **cortex** constitutes lymphoid tissue, while the inner **medulla** contains lymphocytes and discrete clusters of cells, termed *Hassall's corpuscles.* Medullary cells seem to be the principal source of thymic hormones.

Chemistry and metabolism of hormone

In recent years, a number of active principles have been isolated from the thymus which can prevent or reverse the consequences of thymectomy in newborn and adult mammals. Of these, two proteins, **thymosin** with a mol. wt. of less than 10 000 and **thymic humoral factor (thymin)** of mol. wt. less than 6000, have been the subject of most study. Nevertheless, virtually nothing is known of their metabolism and methods of assay are as yet crude and inaccurate.

Action on target tissues

After birth, the development of the capacity to respond to an immunogenic stimulus depends on a functioning thymus gland as well as the other lympho-epithelial tissues of the body. The neonatal thymus gland appears to be essential for the activation and maturation of the rest of the lymphoid defence system involved in 'cellular immunity'. It remains unclear *how* the thymus mediates its effect, but experiments, in which the effects of thymectomy were reversed by thymus grafts contained in cell-impermeable 'diffusion chambers', suggest strongly that a humoral component is involved.

Effects of deficiency

Total thymectomy in neonatal mice results in impaired growth, a reduction in the lymphocyte content of lymphoid organs, immunological unresponsiveness and death. These symptoms can be alleviated by thymus grafts, even within diffusion chambers, or by administration of thymus extracts.

In man, congenital absence or functional depression of the thymus (Di George syndrome) is associated with impaired immunological responsiveness, susceptibility to infection and death within a few months of birth (hypoparathyroidism is also present, see p.15).

Effects of excess

Myasthenia gravis may be associated with thymic hyperplasia in man, but little is known of the effects of deliberate overexposure to thymic hormones in experimental animals.

Control of secretion

The thymus gland interacts with a number of endocrine glands, but, because of the difficulty in assessing directly the rate of thymic hormone secretion, virtually nothing is known of the normal control mechanisms. Growth hormone from the anterior pituitary promotes thymus growth and activity, while, as with other lymphoid tissues, excess adrenal glucocorticoids and ACTH cause atrophy of the thymus. The normal involution of the thymus at puberty appears to be the result of gonadal steroids, since it is prevented by castration.

There is some evidence that abnormal thymus function may be implicated in the pathogenesis of a number of 'auto-immune' diseases such as rheumatoid arthritis, haemolytic anaemia and myaesthenia gravis. In the last condition there is preliminary evidence that a specific thymic factor, termed thymin, may be concerned in the failure of neuromuscular transmission seen in this disease.

Erythropoietin

Erythropoietin is a glycoprotein formed from plasma globulin by the action of a factor from the cortex of the kidney. It stimulates the production of red blood cells by bone marrow.

Chemistry and metabolism of hormone

Erythropoietin is a glycoprotein which has recently been isolated in the pure state: it has a mol. wt. of 23 000. It is formed from a plasma globulin substrate (erythropoietinogen) by the action of an enzyme or enzyme precursor (erythrogenin or renal erythropoietic factor) which is itself released from the

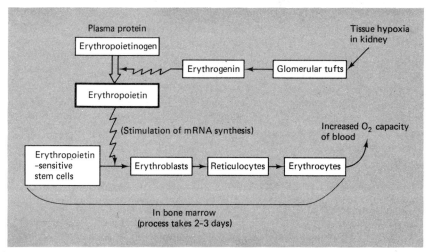

Fig. 10.3 Diagram to illustrate the release and mode of action of erythropoietin.

epithelial cells of the glomerular tufts in the renal cortex (Fig. 10.3) (cf. the renin-angiotensin system discussed on p.135). Erythropoietin is broken down by the liver or excreted in the urine: its plasma half-life is about five hours.

Action on target tissues

Erythropoietin acts on bone marrow and accelerates the maturation of certain (erythropoietin-sensitive) stem cells into erythroblasts. The action of erythropoietin is principally via an increase in RNA synthesis necessary for haemoglobin production.

Effect of deficiency

Chronic renal disease in man is usually accompanied by an anaemia resultant upon impaired erythropoietin secretion. The condition is often reversed after successful renal transplantation.

Effects of excess

Chronic hypoxia in normal subjects as a result of altitude induces an increase in erythropoietin secretion and a consequent increase in the erythrocyte count (erythrocytosis). This condition can also be produced in experimental animals by administration of erythropoietin. Clinically, hypersecretion of erythropoietin and erythrocytosis occurs rarely in chronic renal disease and renal tumours, and very infrequently as the result of erythropoietin-secreting tumours in tissues other than the kidney.

Control of secretion

The rate of erythropoietin secretion is governed by the balance of oxygen supply and oxygen demand in tissues (tissue hypoxia), principally, of course, in the renal cells secreting erythrogenin. Consequently, the usual stimulus to erythropoietin secretion is anaemia, a fall in the Po_2 of blood or perhaps decreased renal blood flow. A number of other factors stimulate erythropoietin secretion; they include androgens, TSH, ACTH, growth hormone, adrenaline; noradrenaline and angiotensin. The physiological significance, if any, of these latter factors to the normal control of erythropoietin secretion remains obscure.

Prostaglandins

Prostaglandins (PG) are twenty-carbon, unsaturated fatty acids which were first demonstrated in the 1930s by the finding that semen contained a smooth muscle stimulant. Since then, some sixteen PG have been characterized. Prostaglandins derive from arachidonic acid (Fig. 10.4) and are conventionally visualized as modifications of a hypothetical precursor, 'prostanoic acid'. Prostaglandin nomenclature is at first sight rather confusing, but is actually a logical shorthand designation of the structural features of the molecule, as shown in Fig. 10.4.

Prostaglandins have been demonstrated in virtually every tissue and are implicated in a wide variety of physiological processes and in most of these appear to modulate cAMP-dependent mechanisms.

There remains a question mark as to whether prostaglandins should be considered to be hormones. Certainly they fail in at least one respect to comply with our definition on p.2, in that most of them are very rapidly metabolized to inactive forms, particularly in the lungs and kidney: this obviously precludes them from any significant role in carrying information *between* tissues. Perhaps they are best considered as local tissue 'hormones' which act by adjusting the final response to signals from conventional hormones and perhaps also from certain nerves.

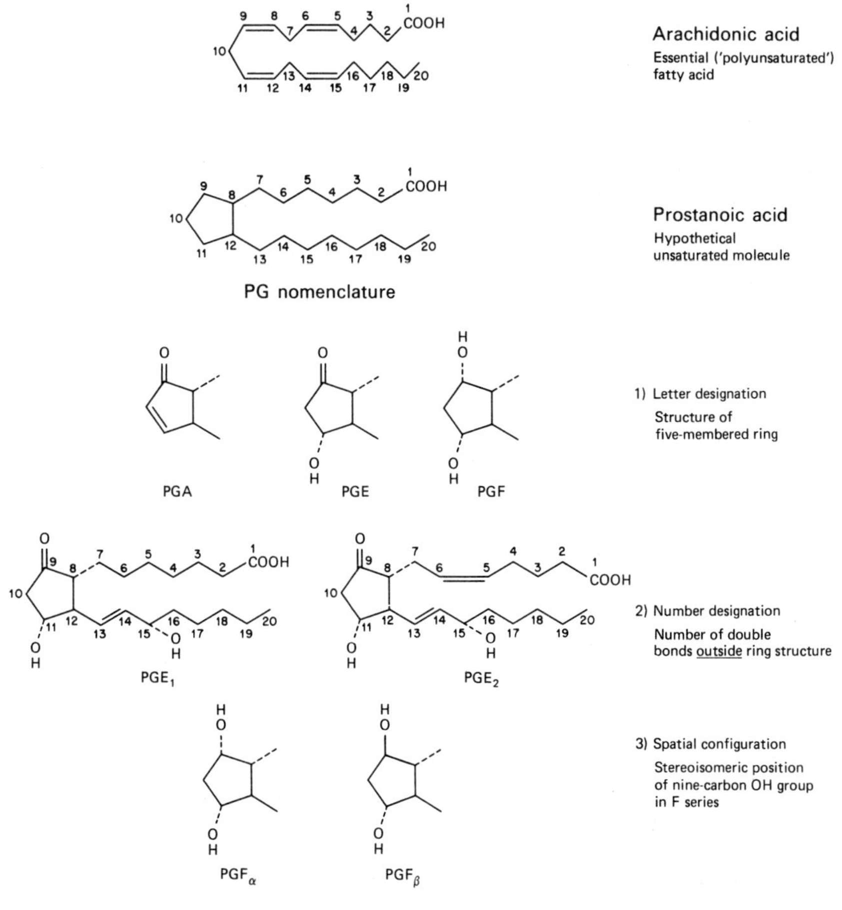

Fig. 10.4 Prostaglandin structure and nomenclature.

It should be noted that much recent attention has been directed towards prostaglandin endoperoxidases and their derivatives, the thromboxanes and prostacylins, by virtue of the multiple biological actions of these substances and, in particular, their possible role in arterial disease.

Further reading

Daggett, Peter (1981). *Clinical Endocrinology*. Edward Arnold, London.

Lands, E. M. (1979). The biosynthesis and metabolism of prostaglandins. *Annual Review of Physiology* **41**, 633.

Nakao, K., Fisher, J. W. and Takaku, F. (Eds.) (1976). *Erythropoiesis*. University Park Press, Baltimore.

Reiter, R. J. (1974). Pineal-anterior pituitary gland relationships. In *Endocrine Physiology*, p.277. Ed. by A. C. Gyton and S. M. McCann. MTP International Review of Science, Physiology, Series I, Vol. 5, Butterworths, London.

Samuelson, B., Granstrom, E., Hamberg, M., Hammarstrom, S. and Malmsten, C. (1978). Prostaglandins and thromboxanes. *Annual Review of Biochemistry* **47**, 321.

Samuelsson, B., Ramwell, P. and Paoletti, R. (Eds.) (1980). *Advances in prostaglandin and thromboxane research*, Vols. 6, 7 and 8. Raven Press, New York.

11

Endocrine control of energy metabolism

'Man ist, was man isst' is a German proverb and pun which means 'one is what one eats'. This is, of course, literally true and provides the theme for this chapter, which is concerned with the hormonal control of the storage and expenditure of metabolic fuel.

It would be an enormous undertaking to attempt to scratch more than the surface of this subject, as is obvious if we review the potential variables involved. These include:

    i. three types of fuel—carbohydrate, fat, protein;

    ii. six hormones—insulin, glucagon, growth hormone, glucocorticoids catecholamines, thyroxine (and T_3);

    iii. four principal tissues—liver, voluntary muscle, brain, adipose tissue;

    iv. a variety of 'challenges' to the regulatory systems—e.g. feeding, fasting, starvation, exercise, cold stress.

No useful purpose would be served in solemnly defining each permutation and combination from the variables above, e.g. the effect of glucagon on carbohydrate metabolism in the muscle of a starving subject. Instead, we will try to construct a general framework for the concept of endocrine regulation of carbohydrate, fat and protein metabolism based on information already outlined in earlier chapters. It is necessary first, however, to examine the extent and nature of the fuel reserves of the body, the daily energy turnover and the requirements of individual tissues.

Fuel reserves

Table 11.1 summarizes the fuel reserve situation in a 70-kg adult male on an adequate occidental diet.

1. It is obvious that fat constitutes the main energy store: there are two main advantages in this. First, fat is the most efficient means of storing energy on a weight basis: fat 40 kJ/g (9.6 kcal/g): carbohydrate and protein 17 kJ/g (4.1 kcal/g). Secondly, the potential storage space for fat has almost unlimited volume, as can be seen in extreme obesity.

2. Only about 0.5 per cent of the reserves is carbohydrate, which represents

Table 11.1 Approximate fuel reserves in an average man

Fuel	Store	kJ	kcal	Percentage of total
Triglyceride	Adipose tissue	420 000	100 000	80
Glycogen	Liver	840	200 ⎫	
	Muscle	1 680	400 ⎬	<0.5
Glucose	Body fluids	170	40 ⎭	
Protein	Mainly muscle	105 000	25 000	20
	Total	527 690	125 640	

less than twenty-four hours supply. Therefore, since the brain *must* have carbohydrate (see p.36), it follows that the supply must be maintained, either from the diet, or by gluconeogenesis.

3. Twenty per cent of the reserves are protein, mainly in muscle. Since most proteins are performing an obvious structural and functional role, they are not readily accessible as routine everyday fuel, but can be called upon after prolonged food deprivation.

In times of plenty, carbohydrate is the preferred energy 'currency', as can be seen from Table 11.2, which shows that it provides about half the daily basal energy requirement, and thus the carbohydrate reserve is 'turned-over' in less than twenty-four hours. The brain can only metabolize glucose (p.36), except in prolonged starvation when ketones can be used, and moreover, although other tissues can use fat, a minimal amount of glucose is required to permit complete oxidation.

In view of the crucial importance of glucose, it is not surprising that the way it is distributed to tissues is closely controlled and that the blood glucose concentration provides a valuable index of energy status. We will, therefore, begin to build up an overall picture of hormonal control of energy metabolism by examining the regulation of blood glucose concentration in terms of a simple hydraulic model (Fig. 11.1).

Table 11.2 Basal daily energy turnover in an average man

	Grams	kJ	kcal	Percentage of total
Carbohydrate	200	3435	820	49
Protein	70	1215	290	17
Fat	60	2413	576	34
Total		7063	1686	

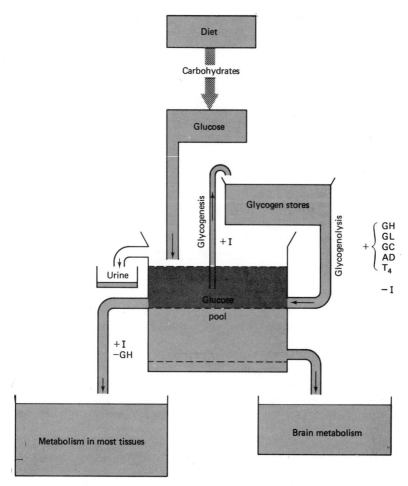

Fig. 11.1 Diagram to illustrate the concept of the blood glucose 'pool' and the processes which influence the size of the 'pool' (see text). Hormones which stimulate (+) or inhibit (−) particular processes are abbreviated thus: I = insulin; GH = growth hormone; GL = glucagon; GC = glucocorticoids; AD = adrenaline; T_4 = thyroxine. (From Hardy, R. N. (1976). *Homeostasis*. Studies in Biology Series. Edward Arnold, London.)

The blood glucose concentration is represented as the level of fluid in a tank, which will clearly depend upon the algebraic sum of the inflow and outflow of glucose. There are two sources of inflow: first, the intermittent addition of glucose to the blood which occurs after meals as the result of the absorption of the carbohydrate in the dict and, secondly, hepatic glycogenolysis. Glucose is lost from the pool as it is utilized by tissues or stored as glycogen and, if the concentration becomes sufficiently high, it can also be lost into the urine. Normally in man, blood glucose concentration remains within the range indicated by the shaded area on Fig. 11.1. Thus, during the absorptive phase after a meal, levels may reach 6.1 to 6.7 mmol/l (110–120 mg glucose/100 ml blood), whereas, after a moderate fast, the concentration may fall to 3.3 to 5.0 mmol/l (60–90 mg/100 ml) Daggett: *Clinical Endocrinology*, Chapter 2). At the upper end of the normal range there is net glycogenesis, i.e. more glucose is being incorporated into glycogen stores than is being released. If the blood glucose concentration falls below about 3.3 mmol/l (60 mg/100 ml), insulin secretion ceases and thus no glucose can enter muscle and adipose tissue cells, which then depend upon fat for their metabolic energy. If the concentration continues to fall (profound hypoglycaemia), insufficient glucose is available even for the brain, and convulsions, coma and death ensue (see Table 4.2).

Regulation of carbohydrate stores

How then are the movements of glucose directed? The answer lies principally in the actions of various hormones which serve as 'flow valves' and regulate appropriately the entry of glucose into cells, glycogenesis and glycogenolysis. Six hormones exert major effects, which are summarized in Fig. 11.1, where + indicates stimulation of a process and – inhibition. Consider first the entry of glucose into cells; this process is insulin dependent in most tissues other than the brain, gut and kidney (p.32). The secretion of insulin is primarily determined by the blood glucose concentration (p.44), such that insulin is not secreted if blood glucose concentration is less than 3.3 mmol/l (60 mg/100 ml), and progressively more insulin is secreted as the glucose concentration increases above this threshold. The consequence of this is that in times of glucose deficit, the little glucose available cannot enter cells whose glucose entry is insulin dependent and it is thus reserved for tissues such as the brain: the other cells have to rely on fat for their metabolic energy. In addition to its effects on glucose entry into cells, insulin stimulates glycogenesis and inhibits glycogenolysis, both of which actions are also directed towards lowering blood glucose concentration (p.32). Insulin, the secretion of which is augmented by increased blood glucose, serves by at least three means to lower blood glucose—negative feedback; it is of vital importance to the regulation of metabolic energy supply, for it is the *only* hormone with hypoglycaemic actions. As can be seen from Fig. 11.1, glucagon, glucocorticoids, adrenaline, growth hormone and thyroxine all stimulate the breakdown of glycogen, while growth hormone slows glucose entry into certain cells. These hormones, therefore, tend to raise blood glucose concentration and, as might be expected, their secretion is stimulated by a fall in blood glucose. There is, therefore, a dual negative feedback control imposed upon blood glucose concentration: hyperglycaemia stimulates insulin secretion, which promotes a hypoglycaemic response, and conversely, hypoglycaemia inhibits insulin secretion while stimulating the release of other hormones with hyperglycaemic actions.

Inter-relations between carbohydrate, fat and protein metabolism

It would be extremely naive to consider the regulation of blood glucose concentration in isolation, as it is so intimately involved with the metabolism

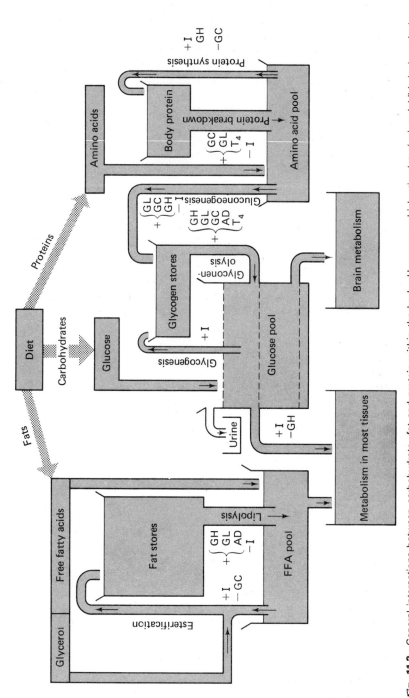

Fig. 11.2 General interactions between carbohydrate, fat and protein metabolism within the body. Hormones which stimulate (+) or inhibit (−) particular processes abbreviated thus: I = insulin; GH = growth hormone; GL = glucagon; GC = glucocorticoids; AD = adrenaline; T₄ = thyroxine. (Modified from Hardy, R. N. (1976). *Homeostasis.* Studies in Biology series. Edward Arnold, London.)

of both fat and carbohydrate. Figure 11.2 attempts to illustrate some of the principal linking pathways.

Fat in the diet is absorbed into the circulation either via the lymphatics as triglycerides, which pass direct into the fat depots, or, after hydrolysis in the gut, as glycerol and free fatty acids (FFA). The FFA pool in the blood comprises FFA absorbed from the gut and FFA released by hydrolysis of triglycerides stored in adipose tissue. The fat stores can be broken down when required by lipolytic enzymes to release FFA into the blood for cellular metabolism. Conversely, in times of plenty, such as after a meal, plasma FFA and glycerol are esterified to replenish the stores. As discussed previously in the case of carbohydrate mobilization, the disposition of fat reserves is again controlled by endocrine 'flow valves', which act by regulating the function of specific enzymes. Figure 11.2 shows that insulin favours and glucocorticoids inhibit the formation of stored fat. Insulin inhibits and growth hormone, glucagon and adrenaline promote lipolysis.

Protein is absorbed from the intestine as amino acids which enter the blood 'pool', from which they can either be taken up by cells and incorporated into protein or converted, via such intermediates as pyruvic acid, into glucose: this latter process is called gluconeogenesis and occurs principally in the liver. Once again, the various pathways are regulated by hormone-controlled 'flow valves', as shown in Fig. 11.2.

It is clear that there is an extremely sophisticated regime of hormones available to mammals to ensure an optimal supply of metabolic energy for the cells of the body. In order to see how the system works in concert, we shall examine the everyday responses to the feeding-fasting cycle.

Effect of feeding

Figure 11.3 summarizes the endocrine responses to feeding, the key to the understanding of which is appreciation of the overwhelming effect of the insulin released. There are a number of factors which promote the secretion of insulin. These are tabulated below and numbered as in Fig. 11.3.

1. Digestion is associated with the secretion of secretin, pancreozymin and a glucagon-like substance from the duodenum: all these hormones stimulate insulin secretion.

2. Activity in the vagus nerve during digestion is thought to cause insulin release in some species.

3. As the products of digestion are absorbed into the blood the increases in (a) glucose concentration, and (b) amino acid concentration both stimulate insulin secretion.

4. Reference to Fig. 11.3 will show that insulin promotes

    a) glucose uptake and utilization by cells;
    b) glycogenesis;
    c) protein synthesis;
    d) esterification.

5. It should be noted that the increased blood glucose concentration tends to depress the secretion of such hormones as glucagon, glucocorticoids, growth hormone and adrenaline.

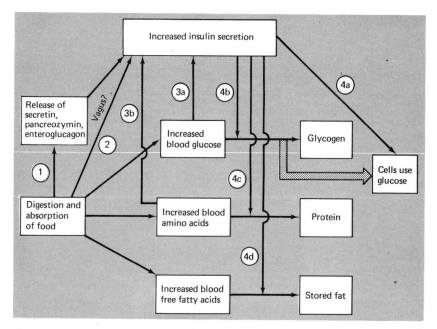

Fig. 11.3 Endocrine and metabolic changes following feeding (see text). (From Hardy, R. N. (1976). *Homeostasis.* Studies in Biology series. Edward Arnold, London.)

Insulin is sometimes called the 'hormone of plenty'. Its copious secretion after meals and the effective way in which it prevents excessive increases in glucose, amino acid and fatty acid concentrations in the blood by promoting their storage at this time, show that this title is amply justified.

Effect of fasting

Figure 11.4 shows the endocrine status after a moderate fast, as in a human subject immediately before breakfast. Once again the figures tabulated below correspond with those in Fig. 11.4. In this situation, the crucial factor is the low blood glucose concentration (hypoglycaemia).

1. Hypoglycaemia depresses insulin secretion.
2. In the relative absence of insulin, glucose uptake by most cells is depressed.
3. The brain does not require insulin for glucose uptake and therefore has the major call on available glucose.
4. Hypoglycaemia stimulates secretion of glucagon, glucocorticoids, growth hormone and, if severe, adrenaline.
5. These hormones stimulate glycogenolysis to maintain entry of glucose into the blood.
6. They stimulate protein breakdown to increase the amino acid pool.
7. They promote gluconeogenesis.

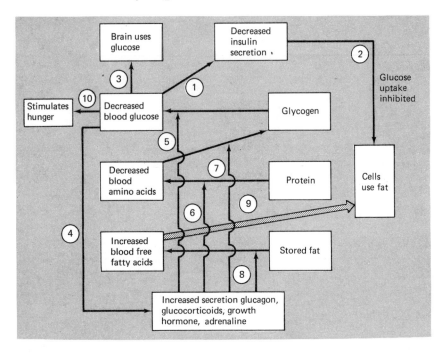

Fig. 11.4 Endocrine and metabolic changes during fasting (see text). (From Hardy, R. N. (1976). *Homeostasis*. Studies in Biology series. Edward Arnold, London.)

8. Perhaps most importantly, they cause breakdown of stored fat.

9. The FFA thus released becomes available to maintain the function of those cells deprived of glucose.

10. Hypoglycaemia stimulates hunger and thus induces the animal to supplement its depleted energy reserves.

These two examples demonstrate the complex way in which the secretion of many hormones may be integrated to ensure that the supply and demand of cellular metabolites maintains a homeostatic balance.

Try now to work out for yourself, using the model developed in Fig. 11.2, how you would expect the system to respond to the demands of (a) exercise, and (b) starvation.

Further reading

Daggett, Peter (1981). *Clinical Endocrinology*. Edward Arnold, London.

Unger, R. H., Dobbs, R. E. and Orci, L. (1978). Insulin, glucagon, and somatostatin secretion in the regulation of metabolism. *Annual Review of Physiology* **40**, 307.

12

Endocrine control of calcium and phosphate metabolism

This chapter attempts to provide an integrated overview of calcium homeostasis by examining first the role of vitamin D_3 and then discussing the interactions of parathormone (PTH), calcitonin (CT) and vitamin D_3 and its derivatives in the control of calcium movement within the body.

Vitamin D

Vitamin D plays an essential role in calcium homeostasis, consequently it must be considered in some detail before any comprehensive discussion of the subject can be undertaken. Vitamin D deficiency gives rise to the characteristic appearance of rickets in children and young animals; skeletal deformities, particularly in the load-bearing bones. Early this century it was found that cod-liver oil contained a substance which prevented rickets and that the condition could also be alleviated by exposure to ultraviolet light. The active principle was named vitamin D (the antirachitic vitamin) and can be formed from either plant or animal dietary precursors (provitamins) by the action of the ultraviolet component of sunlight on the skin (Fig. 12.1) (Daggett: *Clinical Endocrinology*, Chapter 7). Vitamin D_2 will not be considered further, but vitamin D_3 and particularly its hydroxylated derivatives have been shown to manifest a wide variety of actions of fundamental importance to the maintenance of normal calcium balance.

Twenty years ago it was generally thought that vitamin D_3 acted on its target tissues in an unchanged state, but since that time the availability of radioactive vitamin D_3 has allowed a detailed analysis of its metabolism and attention has now focussed on certain of its more biologically active derivatives (Fig. 12.2).

Radioactive vitamin D_3, cholecalciferol (CC), disappears rapidly from the circulation, but in its place a hydroxylated metabolite, 25-hydroxycholecalciferol (25-HCC) appears in the blood. The 25-HCC is formed by the hydroxylation of vitamin D_3 by mitochondrial hydroxylases in the liver: this conversion does not seem to be under ionic or endocrine control. The 25-HCC is bound to a plasma α-globulin and is much more biologically active than the parent vitamin D_3. A further hydroxylation of 25-HCC to 1,25-dihydroxycholecalciferol (1,25-DHCC) may then take place specifically

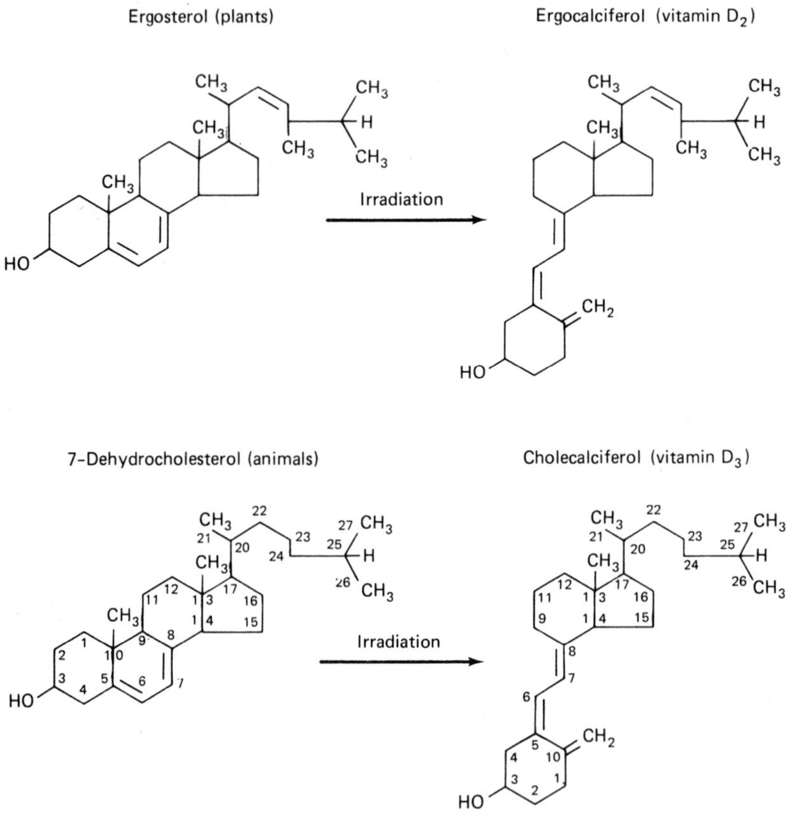

Ergosterol (plants)   Ergocalciferol (vitamin D₂)

Irradiation

7-Dehydrocholesterol (animals)   Cholecalciferol (vitamin D₃)

Irradiation

Fig. 12.1 The structures of vitamin D_2 and vitamin D_3 and their dietary precursors.

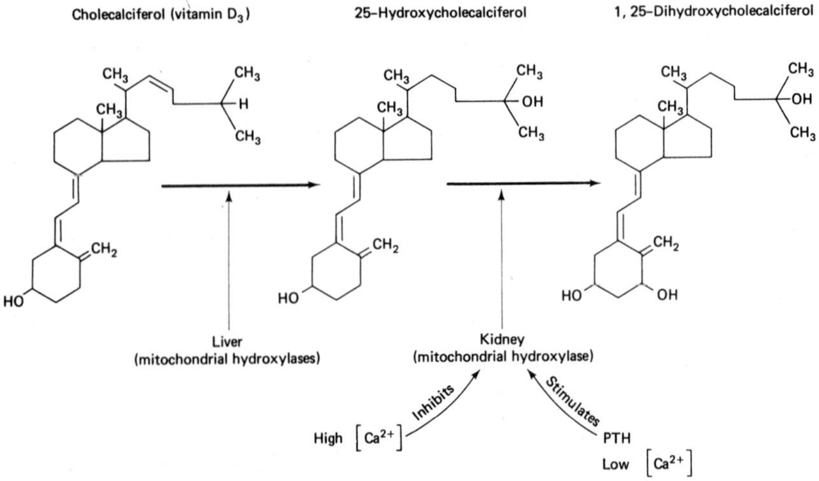

Cholecalciferol (vitamin D₃)   25-Hydroxycholecalciferol   1, 25-Dihydroxycholecalciferol

Liver   Kidney
(mitochondrial hydroxylases)   (mitochondrial hydroxylase)

Inhibits   Stimulates

High $[Ca^{2+}]$ PTH

                                              Low $[Ca^{2+}]$

Fig. 12.2 The hydroxylation of vitamin D_3.

in the kidney. Unlike the conversion of vitamin D_3 to 25-HCC in the liver, the renal hydroxylation of 25-HCC to 1,25-DHCC appears to be dependent upon both ionic and endocrine factors. The evidence remains controversial but, in brief, it seems that the conversion is accelerated in conditions where the extracellular Ca^{2+} concentration is low and inhibited at higher Ca^{2+} concentrations. Moreover, PTH itself seems to stimulate the conversion. Since 1,25-DHCC is much more potent than 25-HCC in terms of facilitating intestinal calcium absorption and the mobilization of bone calcium, it seems entirely appropriate that its production from 25-HCC should be promoted by hypocalcaemia and PTH.

Actions of vitamin D₃, 25-HCC and 1,25-DHCC

Action on intestinal calcium absorption

After administration of vitamin D_3 there is a marked increase in the ability of intestinal epithelial cells to absorb Ca^{2+}. However, this effect is not apparent for a period of several hours and can be shown to result from the production of a specific Ca^{2+}-binding protein in the cells and from the induction of specific ATPases.

> Early work showed that actinomycin D (an inhibitor of protein synthesis) inhibited the action of vitamin D_3 and it was assumed that the actinomycin was inhibiting the effect of the vitamin on the intestinal cells. More recently, however, it has been claimed that the principal action of the inhibitor is on the conversion of 25-HCC to 1,25-DHCC. Certainly, 1,25-DHCC is much more effective than either vitamin D_3 or 25-HCC and its effect on the intestinal cell is not significantly inhibited by actinomycin.

The 1,25-DHCC appears then to be the active principle responsible for the promotion of intestinal absorption of calcium. The sequence of effects is as shown in Fig. 12.3.

a) 1,25-DHCC binds to a specific receptor on the serosal side of the cell.
b) 1,25-DHCC crosses the cytosol and enters the nucleus.
c) 1,25-DHCC initiates nuclear events involving the synthesis of new protein by the polysomes in response to specific mRNA. These events are:
    1) Ca^{2+}-binding protein at the brush border (CaBP).
    2) Ca^{2+}-dependent ATPases at both mucosal and serosal borders, and possibly other enzymes.

As a result of these effects, Ca^{2+} absorption is enhanced by first, facilitating the binding of the ion to the brush border, secondly, pumping it into the cell, and finally, pumping it out into the extracellular fluid.

There is no doubt that the principal importance of vitamin D_3 and its derivatives is upon the intestinal absorption of calcium. However, brief mention must be made of the actions of these substances on bone and kidney.

Action on bone

Vitamin D_3 causes resorption of bone mineral and once again the hydroxylated derivatives, 25-HCC and particularly 1,25-DHCC, are more

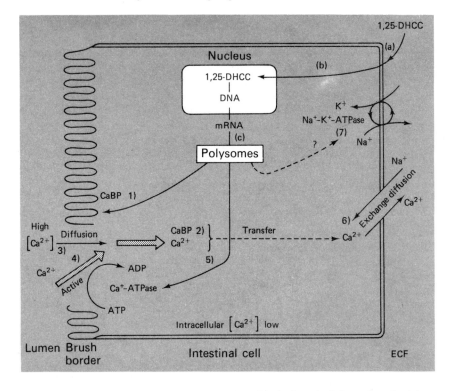

Fig. 12.3 *Scheme to illustrate possible mechanisms for the intestinal absorption of calcium* (see text). (a, b, c) Production of calcium-binding protein (CaBP) from polysomes in response to 1,25-DHCC. CaBP is concentrated at luminal border of cell and may thus facilitate Ca^{2+} uptake (**1**) and/or bind Ca^{2+} once they have entered the cell (**2**) and thereby maintain a low intracellular Ca^{2+}. Because of the low intracellular Ca^{2+}, calcium entry can occur by passive diffusion if the Ca^{2+} in the lumen is high (**3**), but most uptake occurs actively and depends on the presence of a Ca-ATPase produced from the polysomes in response to 1,25-DHCC (**4,5**). Little is known of the mechanisms of Ca^{2+} transfer across the cell: the ion is bound by mitochondria and CaBP. At the serosal border, Ca^{2+} is expelled into the ECF by *exchange diffusion* with Na^+ (**6**). The energy for this process comes indirectly as a result of the low intracellular Na^+ promoted by the Na^+-K^+-ATPase (**7**) which *may* be affected by 1,25-DHCC. NB The rate-limiting step in the sequence is the uptake of Ca^{2+} at the luminal border.

effective than the vitamin itself. The actions of all three agents on bone are blocked by inhibitors of protein synthesis so that their action must involve the production of new protein. The identity and function of this protein remain to be established, but it is known not to be a specific calcium-binding protein.

Action on kidney

Vitamin D_3 and its derivatives probably have little quantitatively significant effect on the renal handling of calcium or phosphate relative to the effects of PTH and CT. However, large doses of vitamin D_3 do have a phosphaturic effect in parathyroidectomized animals.

Calcium balance

Approximately 1.5 per cent of the total body weight is calcium, of which more than 99 per cent is found in the skeleton and teeth, the remainder is found in the extracellular fluid and within the cells.

Since Ca^{2+} plays a vital role in the control of many activities of the body (p.163) it is essential to normal function that the extracellular free Ca^{2+} concentration is regulated within narrow limits. In fact, the free Ca^{2+} concentration of interstitial fluid is closely similar to that in plasma, thus regulation of the free Ca^{2+} concentration in plasma ensures stability throughout the extracellular compartment. However, the free ionized Ca^{2+} in plasma is only a fraction of the total calcium present (Fig. 12.4) (Daggett: *Clinical Endocrinology*, Chapter 7). The remaining calcium is either bound to protein (principally albumin) or in the form of complexes with anions such as phosphate, citrate and bicarbonate. Of these, the complex with phosphate is of particular significance, since phosphate is also involved in the calcification of bone. Thus, increased phosphate levels, by facilitating bone deposition, tend to reduce free Ca^{2+} concentration and, conversely, low phosphate levels are hypercalcaemic. The extent of protein binding is dependent upon the protein concentration and also upon plasma pH; the higher the pH, the greater the protein anion available to bind Ca^{2+}. Free Ca^{2+} concentration is thus, to a certain extent, dependent upon physicochemical factors within the plasma, such as protein concentration, pH and anion status.

Figure 12.5 illustrates the inter-relations between the extracellular calcium pool and the various pathways by which calcium either enters or leaves it.

Total calcium 10 mg/100 ml (2,5 mmol/l)

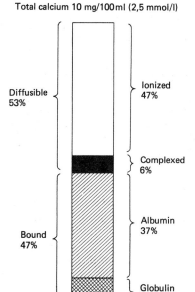

Diffusible 53%

Ionized 47%

Complexed 6%

Albumin 37%

Bound 47%

Globulin 10%

Fig. 12.4 Distribution of serum calcium in adult man.

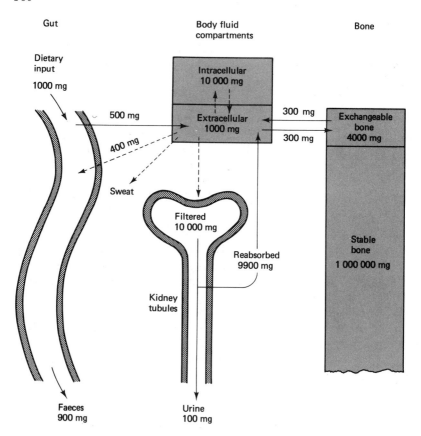

Fig. 12.5 The distribution of calcium in the body. Arrows indicate the direction and magnitude of 24-hour fluxes (see text).

Certain of these pathways, which are shown by broken lines, are not subject to direct control by the factors responsible for calcium homeostasis. These pathways—the exchange between intracellular and extracellular calcium, the glomerular filtration rate, the calcium entering the intestine as an incidental component of gastrointestinal secretions and the small loss in sweat—will not be considered further.

The stability of the extracellular, ionized calcium concentration depends upon a precise balance between the controllable components of input and output. Axiomatically, therefore, the problem resolves itself into equating the input (intestinal absorption + dissolution of labile bone) with the output (renal loss + deposition of bone).

The essentials of the control of the plasma calcium concentration can be embraced within two simple diagrams. Figure 12.6 illustrates the fact, discussed in Chapters 2 and 8, that the rate of secretion of PTH varies inversely and that of CT proportionally with the free Ca^{2+} concentration in plasma.

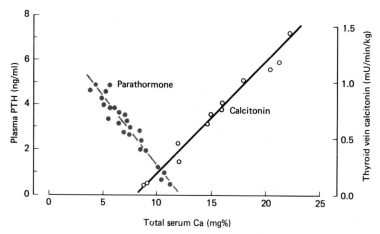

Fig. 12.6 Effects of changes in serum calcium on the concentration of parathormone and calcitonin in peripheral blood. (From Copp, D. H. (1968). Parathyroid hormone, calcitonin and calcium homeostasis. In *Parathyroid Hormone and Thyrocalcitonin (Calcitonin)*, p. 25. Ed. by R. V. Talmage and L. F. Belanger. Excerpta Medica, Amsterdam.)

The pathways by which the secretion of PTH during hypocalcaemia and that of CT during hypercalcaemia serve to maintain the ionized calcium concentration within the normal range are summarized in Fig. 12.7 (the notation of this figure corresponds with the subsequent text).

1. Hypocalcaemia stimulates PTH secretion (and also suppresses CT secretion).

2. PTH acts on labile bone causing the release of Ca^{2+} into the extracellular fluid **A** (p.13) i.e. stimulates osteoclasts.

3. PTH acts on kidney tubules:

a) to depress phosphate reabsorption (phosphaturic effect, p.13) thereby lowering plasma phosphate and promoting bone reabsorption (p.14);
b) to increase Ca^{2+} reabsorption **C** (p.13).

4. PTH probably has a slight facilitatory effect on intestinal absorption of Ca^{2+} (p.14), but its principal influence on this process is an indirect one via (5).

5. PTH accelerates the conversion of 25-HCC to 1,25-DHCC in the kidney (p.157).

6. Vitamin D_3 from the diet has a relatively slight effect on intestinal calcium absorption: 25-HCC has a greater effect.

7. Hypocalcaemia promotes the conversion of 25-HCC to 1,25-DHCC (p.157).

8. 1,25-DHCC is the most important factor in determining the rate of intestinal absorption of Ca^{2+} **B** (p.157).

9. 1,25-DHCC has a slight direct effect on labile bone, promoting resorption and may also act indirectly by enhancing the action of PTH (p.157).

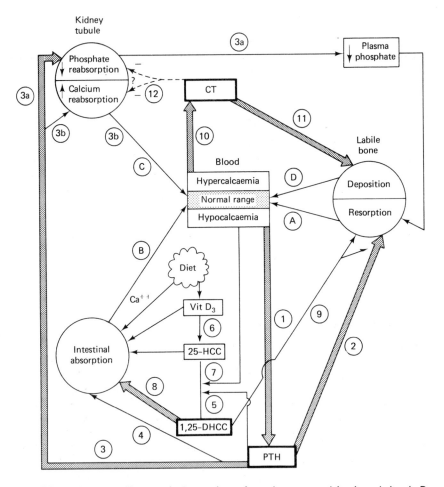

Fig. 12.7 A diagram to illustrate the interactions of parathormone, calcitonin and vitamin D_3 and its derivatives in calcium homeostasis.

The sequence of events described above summarizes the response to hypocalcaemia. During hypercalcaemia, the most important factor that serves to lower the plasma calcium concentration in adult animals is the suppression of PTH secretion, and thus the termination of the mechanisms described under numbers 1–5. In addition, however:

10. hypercalcaemia promotes the secretion of CT;
11. CT favours the incorporation of Ca^{2+} into bone (p.110), thereby lowering blood calcium (D);
12. CT may also have effects on the kidney, although probably not when present at physiological concentrations (p.111).

The hypocalcaemic actions of CT are probably of much more significance in young growing animals than in the adult.

Other hormones concerned in calcium homeostasis

Although PTH, CT and vitamin D_3 and its derivatives are the principal agents responsible for regulating extracellular Ca^{2+} concentration, a number of other hormones can influence the regulatory mechanisms and therefore will be briefly mentioned.

Thyroxine and tri-iodothyronine

Iodinated thyroid hormones stimulate skeletal turnover and bone mineral exchange. Thyroid hyperfunction may therefore be associated with some degree of disturbance of calcium balance. Usually, however, such disturbance is effectively compensated for by the primary regulatory mechanisms.

Sex hormones

Oestrogens favour bone formation; an effect which may involve inhibition of the action of PTH. Androgens stimulate the linear growth of bone and eventually, at the end of adolescence, are involved in the closure of the epiphyses.

Adrenal glucocorticoids

The amounts of cortisol present in the blood under physiological conditions probably exert no significant effects on calcium homeostasis. However, administration of relatively large amounts of cortisol depresses bone formation by inhibiting the synthesis of vital protein and mucopolysaccharide components and also increasing the ratio of osteoclasts to osteoblasts. In addition, in high doses, cortisol decreases intestinal absorption of calcium by inhibiting the hydroxylation of vitamin D_3 to 25-HCC and may also decrease the renal tubular absorption of calcium. Such effects can become important in conditions where overproduction of glucocorticoids occurs (Cushing's syndrome) or where glucocorticoids must be used therapeutically for long periods (collagen diseases).

Growth hormone

The skeleton is one of the major sites of action of growth hormone during active growth. Consequently, it is not surprising that this hormone affects calcium metabolism in several respects. It increases the rate of turnover of bone and also increases both calcium reabsorption from the gut and the renal tubular reabsorption of phosphate: optimal conditions for growth and remodelling of the skeleton thus pertain.

Functions of calcium in the body

The maintenance of a stable extracellular Ca^{2+} concentration is the object of the complex homeostatic mechanisms discussed previously. Such stability is essential since calcium plays a vital part in many aspects of cellular function. Intracellular Ca^{2+} concentration is itself also subject to regulation; thus, despite the tendency for Ca^{2+} to enter the cell down their electrochemical gradient, intracellular concentration is normally low and stable. This is in part due to binding either to specific binding protein or to mitochondria, and in part due to a steady efflux in exchange for other cations, usually Na^{2+} (see Fig. 12.3): alterations in intracellular free Ca^{2+} activity are invariably a prelude or an accompaniment to a change in cellular activity.

Some of the more important functions of Ca^{2+} in the body are listed below.

Structural   Bones, teeth, connective tissue elements, component of intercellular cement substance aiding cell adhesion.

Excitable cells   Functional stability of nerve membranes (see p.14), release of chemical transmitters at nerve endings (e.g. ACh at motor end-plate), excitation–contraction coupling in skeletal muscle, responsible for action potentials in certain types of smooth muscle, involved in action potential and activation of contraction in cardiac muscle.

Endocrine glands   Many examples of Ca^{2+} and cAMP in intracellular regulation of endocrine activity (p.8). Involved in release of exocytosis of stored hormones, e.g. stimulus-secretion coupling in adrenal medulla, (p.19), release of insulin (p.29), anterior pituitary hormones (p.75) and neuro-secretion in the neurohypophysis (p.57).

Exocrine glands   Necessary for the secretion of water and enzymes by the salivary glands and exocrine pancreas and for acid and enzyme secretion by the stomach.

Enzymes   The activity of many enzymes can be shown to depend on the concentration of Ca^{2+}, e.g. the enzyme converting prothrombin to thrombin, thus Ca^{2+} is necessary for blood clotting.

Control of phosphate metabolism

Phosphorus occurs in blood in three major forms, inorganic phosphate, ester phosphate and lipid phosphate. However, the term plasma phosphate conventionally refers only to the inorganic phosphate. Plasma phosphate concentration is more labile than that of calcium and may vary between 2.4 and 4.5 mg/100 ml in the adult (0.8 – 1.5 mmol/l).

Parathormone is the predominant factor in influencing plasma phosphate concentration, but it must be stressed that its influence is not a truly regulatory one, to the extent that changes in phosphate concentration are secondary consequences of the prime role of PTH in the control of plasma calcium. Parathormone mobilizes both calcium and phosphate via the stimulation of bone resorption; however, any tendency for phosphate concentration to increase is counterbalanced by the phosphaturic action of the hormone. Consequently, a parallel increase in calcium and phosphate concentration with the resultant undesirable and dangerous precipitation of calcium phosphate salts is avoided.

Further reading

Daggett, Peter (1981). *Clinical Endocrinology*. Edward Arnold, London.
DeLuca, H. F. (1979). *Vitamin D. Metabolism and Function*. Springer-Verlag, Berlin.
Greep, R. O. and Astwood, E. B. (1976). Endocrinology: Handbook of Physiology, Vol. VIII. *Parathyroid Gland*. American Physiological Society, Washington.
Hancox, N. M. (1972). *Biology of Bone: Biological Structure and Function*, Vol. I. Cambridge University Press, London.
Norman, A. W. (1979). *Vitamin D*. Academic Press, London.

Conclusion

In medieval times it was thought that the four 'humours' (phlegm, blood, bile and black bile) were instrumental to the functioning of the body. If that were indeed the case, then endocrinology would be somewhat simpler and would hardly justify writing or reading this book (as it is we have considered more than forty hormones or similar substances).

However, as a result of work this century, it has gradually become clear that the endocrine system is one of the two great control systems of the body.

Unlike the nervous system, the endocrine system shows great morphological and embryological heterogeneity: thus, some endocrine tissues derive from the gastrointestinal tract (e.g. adenohypophysis, thyroid, pancreas), some from neural ectoderm (e.g. pineal, neurohypophysis, adrenal medulla), while yet others come from mesodermal origins (e.g. adrenal cortex, gonads). Nevertheless, the basic elements of endocrine secretion discussed in Chapter 1 remain common to all.

During evolution, hormones and endocrine systems have either adapted their function to new circumstances or disappeared. Thus, insulin is present in fish to regulate amino acid metabolism, while in man this function has become overshadowed by its influence on carbohydrate and fat metabolism. On the other hand, urotensin is a fish hormone which is secreted by the urophysis and is concerned in osmoregulation; both gland and hormone presumably found no place in the physiology of terrestrial animals and have thus disappeared.

Paradoxically perhaps, in some respects one of the most exciting ways ahead in endocrinology concerns the past; in such fields as the evolutionary hierarchy of brain/pituitary/placenta peptides alluded to in Table 7.4, and the brain/gut peptides mentioned in Chapters 5 and 7 and their phylogenetic inter-relations. A deeper assessment of these areas could do much for our understanding of the links between nervous and endocrine systems and, in so doing, provide a great deal of information of potential clinical importance.

Index

Index